Back Pain

Solutions

How to Help Yourself with Posture-Movement Therapy and Education

Bruce I. Kodish, Ph.D., P.T.

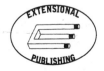

EXTENSIONAL PUBLISHING

Pasadena, CA

Back Pain Solutions
by Bruce I. Kodish
Copyright © 2001 by Bruce I. Kodish

Published by Extensional Publishing
            Post Office Box 50490
            Pasadena, CA 91115-0490
            Fax: 626-441-2339
            Telephone: 626-441-4627
            Email: ExtensionalPubl@aol.com

Publisher's Catalogue in Publication Data
Kodish, Bruce I.
Back Pain Solutions / by Bruce I. Kodish
Pasadena, CA:Extensional Publishing, © 2001
320 pp. includes index
ISBN 0-9700664-5-7 (paperback: alk. paper)
Library of Congress Card Number: 00–191164

1. Backache. 2. Physical Therapy. 3. Physical Education and Training.
4. Posture. 5. Pain. 6. Alexander Technique. 7. Mechanical Diagnosis
and Therapy.
I. Title. II. Kodish, Bruce I.

LC Classification # RD771.B17
Dewey Decimal Classification # 617.564

Cover Design by Edward Dawson
Illustrations/Drawings by Max Sandor and Bruce I. Kodish

Disclaimer:
Every effort has been made to make the information in this book as complete and as accurate as possible. However, new information may become available after the printing date. In addition, mistakes, both typographical and substantive may have occurred. Therefore this text should be used only as a general guide. You are urged to read other available material. The publisher and author expressly disclaim any and all liability or responsibility to any person or entity for any injury, loss or harm of any kind, directly or indirectly caused or alleged to be caused from the use of the ideas and information contained in this book. If you have or develop any adverse symptoms you need to consult an appropriate healthcare professional for diagnosis and possible contraindications. See Chapter 8 for guidelines to determine when to see a physician. **If you do not wish to be bound by this disclaimer, you may return this book to the publisher for a full refund.**

For more information go to www.backpainsolutions.net
You may contact the author at backsolutions@aol.com

Contents

When you're hungry, sing; when you're hurt, laugh.
– Jewish Proverb[1]

Dedication

I dedicate this book to my parents. My mother of beloved memory, Dorothy Berson Kodish, often reminded me to "act like a mensh!"[1] I'm happy that some of her directness, spontaneous humor and creativity rubbed off on me—at least I think it did. She consistently encouraged me by letting me know that I could stand up for myself and do what I set out to do. My father, Morris 'Mashe' Kodish, has demonstrated throughout his life a quiet competence—with some swearing—that has shown me what it means to do what needs doing. I admire his toughness and independence and am grateful for his humor and love. Both my parents helped me develop a Grade-A 'crap detector', gave me my love of books and showed me that self-reliance and the love of learning depend on your attitude and not on your title or on what degrees you have.

I am also grateful to my uncle, Sam Berson, who encouraged me with his quiet humor to think for and challenge myself. I miss him. My deep gratitude also goes to my in-laws, Beatrice and George Samuelson, who supported me throughout the development of my career. I miss their wit and courage.

I also feel gratitude to all of my physical therapy teachers (including fellow students) at the University of Pittsburgh and elsewhere. I feel a debt as well to my Alexander Technique teachers, in particular Troup Mathews—who showed me what "growing young" means—and Ann Mathews and Christine Batten, for their patient teaching of a sometimes unruly student.

I feel indebted to my many students, patients and clients over the years for helping me to learn what I could not get from books or teachers.

Finally, I owe a debt to the work of Alfred Korzybski, perhaps best known for his statement, "A map is not the territory." This book may be seen as my application of General Semantics, the discipline which Korzybski founded, to the problem of back pain. My deep gratitude goes to all of my teachers and colleagues at the Institute of General Semantics. In particular, Charlotte Schuchardt Read and Robert P. Pula have helped me to apply a scientific attitude (extensional orientation) to my own life. I'm still working at it.

Acknowledgements

I wish to thank all those who read one or more versions of the manuscript and contributed with critiques, comments and discussion. These include Ron Dennis, Ed.D.; Barrett Dorko, P.T.; Gary Jacob, D.C.; Marilyn Kodish Sutherland; Rick Marken, Ph.D.; Max Sandor, Ph.D.; and Kristi Pallino. My wife Susan Presby Kodish, Ph.D., served as chief editor. Without her critical eye, love and untiring support I could not have produced this book.

Preface:
Who Is This Book For?

Welcome to *Back Pain Solutions*! If you are currently experiencing back pain, you have taken an important step to learning how to reduce and abolish your symptoms.

If you've had one or more episodes of back pain, this book is also for you. Time may not heal all wounds. If you've been left with some residual pain, disability and fear of recurrence, techniques in this book can help you find the confidence you need to move through life with greater ease.

Even if you are not concerned about back pain, you will find something of value here if you want to improve your posture and efficiency of body use. You can also share this book with someone you care about who is dealing with back pain. The self-care principles I discuss apply to neck pain, repetitive strain and other joint and muscle pains, as well.

The opportunity to feel better is there for those who understand the possibilities of self-care for back and related pain problems. These possibilities have been understood and available for many years but have been mostly unknown to the general public and much of the medical community.

This book can also help medical doctors, physical therapists, chiropractors, massage therapists, body workers and movement educators to learn some new and different ways of helping themselves and the people with whom they work.

I have attempted to be reasonably comprehensive. Nonetheless, this book offers *some* back pain solutions, not 'the' solution or 'all' solutions. When possible, I point out where to go for more help and further information. In the Notes section at the end of the book, I provide references and technical comments. For ease of reference, I have numbered those places in the text that have a note.

I will be very surprised if you cannot find at least one thing in this book to help your condition to some degree. Look for small improvements. Small changes can lead to big differences in some unexpected ways.

Bruce Kodish
Pasadena, CA
January, 2001

Usage Note:
To avoid confusion, I here explain my varying uses of double and single quotes throughout the book. I apply double quotes according to standard usage to indicate both direct quotes and terms/phrases used by someone but not necessarily indicating a direct quote. I use single quotes in the standard way to indicate a quotation within a quotation. I also use single quotes to mark off terms and phrases which seem in varying degrees misleading (see *Drive Yourself Sane* for further explanation). The single quotes here serve as a safety device to alert the reader to take care when using such terms. For example, using terms such as 'mind', 'body', etc., may mislead one into assuming that what corresponds to each term exists in the non-verbal world as an isolated, separate entity. I also use single quotes to mark off terms used metaphorically or playfully.

My use of such language as "some," "to me," "as I see it," "seem(s)," "to some degree," etc., may seem too indefinite or "wishy-washy" for some readers. I do not apologize. Rather, this represents my conscious effort to use an approach to language called EMA, English Minus Absolutism, which was formulated by General Semantics writer Allen Walker Read. As Read has said, " It is clear to many of us that we live in a process world, in which our judgements can only be probabilistic. Therefore we would do well to avoid finalistic, absolutistic terms. Can we ever find 'perfection' or 'certainty' or 'truth'? No! Then let us stop using such words in our formulations."[1]

Introduction

Thought is born of failure.
- L. L. Whyte[1]

Chapter 1

Is It Possible To Feel Better?

You wake up one morning feeling stiff in your back. "What did I do?" you wonder. You drag yourself out of bed...carefully. No, this isn't just a stiff back; *it hurts*. You feel a twang of pain which catches you if you move too quickly. It goes across your back and into your butt on one side. Bending over the sink to wash is a mistake. Ouch!

Despite being as careful as you think you can be, the pain persists for the next few days. You try to figure out what caused it but can't be very sure. Was it that gardening the other day? Your back did feel kind of stiff after you were bending over for an hour pulling weeds. Hmm. What is wrong? You begin to worry, "Should I go to the doctor?" Or maybe you already have gone to the doctor, who has reassured you that nothing serious is wrong, that this too shall pass. And it does—mostly it does—but perhaps not as much as you'd like. And perhaps you wonder when another episode will strike and whether there isn't something more that you can do to prevent it.

If your back hurts, you may have already tried various types of treatment with varying effects. However, if you felt entirely satisfied, you probably wouldn't be reading this, would you?

The field of back pain treatment is filled with multiple professions making conflicting diagnoses, presenting confusing claims and offering contradictory-seeming care with sometimes questionable results.

When practitioners offering treatments continue to debate and fail to agree upon "Where is the pain coming from?" and "What can be done about it?" how do you, someone with back pain, decide what to believe and to whom to go to for help?

Back pain can have multiple causes. Some of the apparent confusion may have to do with the fact that effectively treating this common complaint provides greater problem-solving challenges than many people realize.

For example, one source of confusion comes about because any particular episode of back pain tends to run its course, with the sufferer feeling better, if not completely pain-free, with the passage of time alone. How then can you judge whether a treatment offers real benefits or simply allows you to fool yourself into thinking that it does?

Another reason for the continuing and confusing diversity of viewpoints about back pain comes from the explosive growth of medical information. This has made it easier for genuinely useful knowledge to get buried and forgotten.

In this book I present some ways to help you cut through the confusion. While further research is needed, some sound and practical methods already exist for helping you to reduce, eliminate and prevent your back pain symptoms.

Posture-Movement Therapy and Education

Back Pain Solutions is based on the simple, far-reaching and widely-agreed-upon insight stated by Dr. Gordon Waddell in his book, *The Back Pain Revolution*: " Back pain is a mechanical problem in the sense that symptoms arise from the musculoskeletal system and vary with physical activity."[1] In this book, I will use the terms "mechanical" and "activity-related" interchangably to refer to this type of pain.

Back pain researchers have long understood common, everyday back pain as mechanical.[2] Dr. Richard Deyo, a noted researcher on the subject, has written that as much as 98% of back problems comes under the category of activity-related pain.[3] However, the practical implications of this understanding have yet to become common knowledge to many people with back pain.

Activity-related (mechanical) back pain varies with activity. Such activity includes changes in posture and movement. *Back Pain Solutions* is based upon my study of a number of therapeutic and educational approaches that explore the relations of posture and movement to human functioning. I have integrated these approaches into a two-tiered framework that I call *Posture-Movement Therapy and Education.*

Posture-Movement Therapy

The first tier of activity-related solutions for back pain is *posture-movement therapy.* Posture-movement therapy includes the relatively short-term use of static postures (positions) and movements to ameliorate pain, other symptoms and loss of movement. If you have mechanical (activity-related) pain, you may be able to influence it through the application of specific positions and movements applied as exercises. You may be able to do this on your own or with coaching as needed. This insight has been especially developed in detail by physical therapist Robin McKenzie and his colleagues.[4]

Positions and movements can also be guided, facilitated or passively applied in the form of manipulative or manual therapy by an experienced practitioner. Manipulative techniques exist on a continuum with the previously noted exercises. My own bias is to first see what individuals can do for themselves with the necessary coaching. However, positions and movements applied by a hands-on practitioner may have great usefulness as well.

Health professionals who offer one or more kinds of such activity-related treatment include physical therapists, chiropractors, osteopaths and medical doctors specializing in manual medicine. Many different schools of thought within each of these specialties exist. Different practitioners may have different theories and use different approaches and techniques. Interestingly enough, despite these differences there also exists a great deal of overlap and similarity. This also holds true for different educational methods which I'll discuss in the next section.

Nonetheless, different terms for similar things or the same terms for differing things can lead to confusion and unnecessary opposition. The profusion of theories, terminology and techniques can seem daunting. I offer the term "*posture-movement*" as a neutral, descriptive label for the many varying approaches to therapy and education.

The term "mechanical therapy and education," which could label such approaches, has lost its neutrality because it has become too closely identified with one particular school of thought, the "Mechanical Diagnosis and Therapy" of Robin McKenzie. Although I value it enough to have studied and become certified in it, I recognize that this approach does not include the full range of activity-related methods available. Also, the term 'mechanical' can have a machine-like connotation that some people may find off-putting.

"Activity-related treatment and education," which I use at times, provides a more neutral term but lacks a certain descriptiveness.

The term "posture-movement" labels in a descriptive and easily understandable way the kinds of problems dealt with and the types of solutions provided. It indicates the relations between posture and movement. (See The Problem with Posture in the next chapter.) It does not refer to any particular or 'patented' approach. I offer it, rather, as a unifying term that different practitioners can use to talk about the commonalities of what they do.

It can refer to both therapy and education approaches. What distinguishes posture-movement therapy from posture-movement education? Posture-movement *therapy,* as I define it, is practiced by a properly trained and duly licensed healthcare professional. Someone offering posture-movement therapy should have the ability to diagnose or screen for non-mechanical problems that may require referral for appropriate medical or surgical care. The practitioner should also be trained to offer activity-related (posture-movement) treatment that directly deals with specific pain and other symptoms through the use of activity-related assessment, the use of specific exercises and/or manipulative treatments, and the ongoing assessment of the effects of treatment.

Posture-Movement Education

Many have noted the effects of posture on human performance and functioning. In relation to pain, your everyday postural habits—how you typically sit, stand, bend, lift, walk, move, etc.—may influence activity-related symptoms.

Posture-movement education is the second tier of activity-related solutions for back pain. It focuses on the improvement of your everyday posture-movement habits—your learned, mostly automatic postural behavior. Posture-movement education in itself is not a therapy. It does not in itself involve the diagnosis, screening or treatment of specific pain problems. Posture-movement education involves more long-term and indirect preventive instruction.

In understanding the role of posture, I particularly draw upon the principles and methods of the Alexander Technique of Psycho-Physical (Cognitive-Kinesthetic) Education.[5] The Alexander Technique (AT) focuses on the application of conscious thought (Cognition) and sensory perception of the body (Kinesthetic awareness) to improve posture and performance. Ronald J. Dennis, Ed.D., a researcher and teacher of the Alexander Technique, defines it simply as "a nonexercise approach to the improvement of body mechanics."[6]

Besides the Alexander Technique, which I was trained in, there are many other educational approaches that can address your habits of posture and movement. These include Body

Harmony, the Feldenkrais method, Ideokinesis, Rolfing, Sensory Awareness, Simple Contact, and the Trager Approach, among others.[7] Studies in these approaches as well as in applied anatomy, body mechanics and ergonomics, have enriched my thinking and practice.

A point of clarification: Both posture-movement therapy and posture movement education exist along a continuum. Many healthcare practitioners who offer therapy also place a major emphasis on education for back pain and other problems. Educational methods such as the Alexander Technique (practiced by qualified teachers), though not therapies themselves, may lead to therapeutic effects for those who study them.

This book will provide basic information that you need in order to recognize whether you have a mechanical (activity-related) problem. The combination of posture-movement therapy and posture-movement education reveals principles that work together in a unique and synergistic way. You can then begin to explore how to use both exercises and posture as self-help tools to find your own back pain solutions.

A Scientific Attitude

In order to make the best use of the self-help tools discussed in this book, I suggest that you consider yourself as a personal scientist.[8] As a personal scientist you can apply a scientific attitude, not only in those subject areas that you think of as 'science', but also in your everyday life and problem-solving. A scientific attitude involves an open-minded examination of your assumptions, with a willingness to test and revise them on the basis of available evidence.

You can follow these steps as you apply the self-help methods for activity-related pain that I discuss in this book:

• Clarify your problem. This can include uncovering your assumptions about the problem and about possible solutions.

• Ask answerable questions based on these assumptions.

• Make observations in a calm, unprejudiced manner to answer these questions.

• Report your observations to yourself, and perhaps others, as accurately as possible and in such a way as to answer the questions that you asked to begin with.

• Revise your assumptions as necessary in light of the observations made and the answers obtained.

• Cycle through the process again and again.

As a scientific explorer in your daily life, you can actually begin with any one of these steps.[9]

The Method of Possibilities

To take such a broad scientific approach to your back problem you don't necessarily need to do formal scientific research with large groups of people, complicated statistics and elaborate analysis. In studying your possibilties for feeling and moving better, you are studying a single case—yourself.

Many researchers pooh-pooh the usefulness of studying single cases, which they call "anecdotal evidence." It is true that if you are trying to generalize about what proportion of a large group of people will respond to a form of treatment, studying one individual will not get you very far. If that is what you are trying to do, recognize that, as an old Jewish proverb says, " 'For example' is no proof."[10]

However, there is another equally accurate Jewish proverb, "We cannot learn everything from general principles; there may be exceptions."[11] One individual, a single case, *can* indicate that something is possible for that individual and perhaps for other individuals as well.

Social science researcher Philip J. Runkel has proposed a name for scientific methods that study the behavior of individuals. He calls such methods "specimen testing." One particular method of specimen testing has special relevance to you. Runkel calls it "the method of possibilities."

The method of possibilities seeks to answer the question, "What can be done?" As Runkel puts it, the method of possibilities involves "a trial of a course of action to find out whether it might be possible to bring it off."[12]

It seems likely that you have not exhausted the possibilities of dealing with your back pain. You can learn to use a scientific approach to explore your back problem and reduce and/or eliminate your pain. We will start this exploration in the next chapter with a look at the personal and social costs of back pain.

Part I
Problems and Solutions

Almost anything is easier to get into than out of.
- Agnes Allen[1]

Chapter 2

Back Pain Problems

"She killed herself," a friend of mine told me of a co-worker. "After years of chronic back pain, multiple surgeries and heavy pain medication, she had had enough."

This kind of tragedy fortunately doesn't happen very often. Much more likely, a person with chronic or recurrent back pain just learns to "live with it." When her back 'goes out', she restricts her activities, may take time off from work and, with medication, a certain amount of grit, and whatever other form of therapy she chooses, waits it out. Does this sound familiar?

Karen

The frustration experienced by those with persistent back pain is apparent in what happened to one person I worked with.[1]

Karen, a young woman in her early thirties, had over a decade of activity-related back troubles. Over these years, she saw many different kinds of health professionals. She had x-rays, MRI (Magnetic Resonance Imagery) and other tests and received many different diagnostic labels for her recurring problems. Treatments she received included pain medication, hot packs, electrical stimulation, spinal manipulation and exercises. During these years she had four particularly bad episodes during which time she was briefly hospitalized and then placed on extended bed rest.

After one such recurrence she went to an orthopedic surgeon who neither looked at her back nor examined her. After hearing some of her history, he said, "Why haven't you had your disc removed?"

"What's the alternative?" she asked.

"*Whining* for the *Rest* of your *Life*," he replied.

She did not return to his office.

At various times Karen also saw a number of chiropractors. While adjustments (the chiropractic term for spinal manipulation) sometimes seemed to help for brief periods,there were times when they didn't help or seemed to make her worse. Chiropractic adjustments, she found, could be applied in the same rote way as some of the other treatments she had gotten from physicians and therapists. Some chiropractors she met also emphasized returning for frequent and periodic adjustments, even when she didn't experience a problem.

Following each episode, Karen often got advice to stay active, do exercises and work on her posture. However, typically she would be handed a few stapled sheets of paper with generic instructions. Occasionally, she was given more personalized attention, not all of it helpful.

During one episode when she experienced pain in both her back and leg, a physician showed her an exercise he wanted her to do. As she lay flat on her back, she was instructed to pull one knee to her chest. After several repetitions, the pain in her leg increased and shot down into her foot. "Try not to pay any attention to it," he told her as the pain in her foot increased. She finally stopped the exercise, in tears.

She recalls a more positive experience when a physical therapist patiently answered her questions and worked with her on the exercises he gave her. The therapist got into trouble for the extra time he spent with her. On her next visit, she was treated by someone else.

She became resolved to "live with my problem" until, by a set of chance circumstances, she came to see me.

Back Pain Problems

Back pain is common. It ranks as the fifth most likely reason for visiting a medical doctor.[2] As many as 80% of adults can expect to experience back pain at some time in their lives.[3] In any one year, 56% of adults will probably experience some back pain while 18% will have frequent episodes within that year's time and 15% will experience back pain lasting more than 30 days.[4] Although Karen belongs to the smaller category of people with frequent or chronic pain, her story illustrates some of the difficulties confronted by anyone with a significant back problem.

The Diagnostic Daze

The majority of back problems are, like Karen's, activity-related, involving some transient injury to the moving parts of the spine (muscles, joints, ligaments and discs). Yet it appears that the actual parts of the back responsible for such mechanical pain are often difficult, if not impossible, to determine with any accuracy.[5]

In their efforts to come up with a diagnosis, some practitioners may give too much credence to x-rays and other kinds of diagnostic imagery that do not always correlate neatly with the symptoms that people experience. By now, many studies have been done that show a significant lack of correlation between symptoms experienced and what one sees on diagnostic imaging.[6,7] Among a group of people who reported never having had back pain, about 20% had herniated discs according to MRI studies. Of this same group, about 50% of those under 60 and almost 80% of those over 60 had bulging discs.[8]

This does not mean that arthritic changes or a bulging or herniated disc can never cause back pain. It does mean that having these visible problems on your x-ray or MRI does not necessarily mean that you will have pain.

In addition, many of the other potentially problematic parts of the back cannot be seen on x-rays or MRI images, or detected with laboratory tests. Diagnosis and treatment should not be based solely on imaging results. People like Karen may become unduly frightened by practitioners who conclude more than they ought to from such tests.

For physicians and other health-professionals, who want to know what specific part of the spine is affected, these diagnostic difficulties can seem particularly frustrating. Once serious disease or surgical emergencies (often much easier to detect) are eliminated, we are left with what has come to be called "non-specific back pain," which accounts for the majority of all episodes.

Despite these diagnostic problems, many different groups of practitioners have made an effort to explain as well as they can what happens when someone's back hurts. Different explanations may imply different treatments. There are a variety of approaches, not all of which seem compatible. As Karen discovered, the diagnosis that a person with back pain ends up with may depend more upon whom she has seen than on anything else.[9]

Chiropractors may diagnose "subluxations." Rheumatologists may diagnose "arthritis," internists "low back muscle strains," orthopedists "herniated discs." Might all of these diagnoses be equally correct? Or might all of them be more or less wrong? If there is some 'truth' to at least some of them some of the time, how much and in what way?

Even though, or perhaps *because,* any one practitioner or group of practitioners may show a great deal of assurance in their particular viewpoint, the area of back care as a whole teems with diagnostic and explanatory confusion. As a result, people like Karen often feel confused as well.

Questioning Traditional Treatments

At the worst of her most serious bouts of pain, Karen was hospitalized and then placed on lengthy bed rest, with a focus on receiving passive therapy with treatments like heat packs, cold packs and electrical stimulation. This represented the traditional conventional 'wisdom' which highlighted resting to promote recovery.

For years, a few lonely voices challenged this emphasis on rest in treating back pain. For example, in a 1947 article in the *British Medical Journal* entitled "The Dangers of Going to Bed," R. A. J. Asher wrote, "It is my intention to justify placing beds and graves in the same category and to increase the amount of dread with which beds are usually regarded...There is hardly any part of the body which is immune to its dangers."[10]

More recently, the number of questioning voices has grown. By now, numerous studies have challenged the importance of bed rest as a significant treatment for back pain and sciatica (back pain which radiates into the leg).[11] It is now more widely understood that unduly restricting activities with enforced bed rest can lead to further problems of immobility and disuse.[12] These days, Karen would not be advised to stay in bed so long!

The other widely applied passive treatments that Karen received, such as heat, ultrasound and electrical stimulation, although they may temporarily ease symptoms, have also been de-emphasized. As the Agency for Health Care Policy and Research (AHCPR) guidelines panel noted in their 1994 report, "The use of physical agents and modalities in the treatment of acute low back problems is of insufficiently proven benefit to justify their cost. As an option, patients may be taught self-application of heat or cold to the back at home."[13]

Someone like Karen probably benefits now from another growing trend: reduced willingness to do surgery. Back surgery rates in the United States have been among the highest in the industrialized world. When "failed back surgery" became a diagnosis in its own right, some people began to wonder if these higher surgical rates did equal better healthcare. Despite the attitudes of a few surgeons like the one that Karen met, surgery now has a much smaller role in treatment than previously thought. This leads to more options for the person with back pain, as well as better results when surgery does seem necessary.

Karen's experiences with chiropractic treatment represents the experience of many as well. 40% of those getting care for back pain see a chiropactor.[14] As Karen discovered, spinal manipulation (movements applied to the joints by a practitioner) can sometimes provide relief. Some research evidence indicates that such treatment can provide short-term benefits.

However, as Karen discovered, the long term benefit of such care is not clear. Her confidence was not encouraged by practitioners she met who used this approach as the major part of their treatment and encouraged her to return again and again for adjustments.

When Time Doesn't Heal All Wounds

It has become widely accepted that activity-related back pain has a self-limiting nature. In other words, a person will likely recover from a particular episode simply with the passage of time. According to one widely referenced research study, 44% of those with low back pain were better in a week, 86% were better in a month and 92% in two months.[15]

Therefore, pain medication as necessary, combined with "watchful waiting," appears to some practitioners as the best overall approach for treating this common condition. Watchful waiting involves the person with back pain remaining as active as possible while letting nature take its course.[16]

The expense of dealing with back pain is staggering. By the end of the twentieth century, lost productivity cost U.S. industry more than $28 billion dollars per year. The added costs of disability payments and medical costs may have brought the total loss to more than $50 billion dollars in the U.S. alone.[17] For the sufferer, the expense of continuing or recurring pain involves, in addition to monetary loss, discomfort and emotional distress.

Is watchful waiting and encouraging general activity enough to deal with this epidemic of disability? Is passage of time sufficient?

As Karen learned, she was indeed likely to improve somewhat from any particular episode. However, afterwards she still experienced some pain, restriction and weakness. Having had a series of episodes over many years, she expected future disabling recurrences as well. What then did "getting better" mean?

Although some authorities still seem to believe that most patients recover quickly and spontaneously from an episode of back pain, evidence belies this. Researchers in Great Britain found that a much larger percentage of patients than expected had continuing severe symptoms a year after onset.[18] Israeli researchers found that although the back patients they studied did improve over time, most of them continued having some pain and functional limitations at a two-month follow-up.[19]

Recurrence of back pain also remains a persistent and widely recognized problem.[20] It may be true that for some people each episode will be similar with similar periods of recovery. Unfortunately there is little evidence that everyone can expect full recovery with typical present-day treatment.

For a significant minority of people, ongoing symptoms remain. Some of those who have gotten at least some relief, may have continuing and worsening recurrences. Some develop sciatica, which can include lower limb pain, tingling, numbness and weakness in the muscles of the leg. This syndrome is commonly preceded by recurring episodes of back pain.

Back pain is not necessarily as transient or as self-limiting as it is often presented to be. As Karen learned, passage of time is not always sufficient.

Activity and Exercise

Karen was told to stay as active as possible and encouraged to engage in moderate exercise after her acute episodes. This advice follows the change in conventional wisdom I

discussed earlier. Rest is out. Activity is in. Most practitioners presently agree that enforced and prolonged inactivity
does little good for back pain. Statistical evidence does indicate that, in general, returning to normal activity as quickly
as possible seems beneficial to most people with an acute episode of back pain. Meanwhile, studies of people with chronic
back pain indicate that many seem generally to benefit from
fitness exercises even if they experience some pain while
doing them.[21]

But what activity and exercises are best for an individual?
Some practitioners seemed to have a theoretical rationale for
telling her to do one thing or another. Some doctors told Karen
that, as long as she kept active, no particular exercise seemed
best.[22] When it came down to actually doing exercises, Karen
was often given generic exercises with only vague guidelines
about when to continue in spite of pain or when to stop because of it.

Karen's confusion about exercise reflects the state of research on exercise and back pain. Different theories may explain why an exercise should work or why an activity is useful or harmful to the back. These theories may or may not be
sound. How can anyone know?

Based on their survey of various statistical studies, the
British Royal College of Physicians stated this in its *Clinical
Guidelines for the Management of Acute Low Back Pain:* "On
the evidence available at present, it is doubtful that specific
back exercises produce clinically significant improvements
in acute low back pain or that it is possible to select which
patients will respond to which exercises."[23]

This vagueness and skepticism regarding exercise as well
as other forms of back treatment results in part because much
of modern healthcare has become overly dependent on a
particular, narrow, view of research.

A growing number of healthcare practitioners advocate
what they call 'evidence'-based practice. It seems ironic that

some advocates of this approach emphasize the usefulness of only one form of evidence: information gained from the statistical study of large groups of people.

This kind of information can be useful for making correlations between types of treatment and general outcomes for groups of people. If you want to know whether a particular treatment works on the average, you need this kind of study.

However, there is information that can never be gotten from doing this kind of research. Statistical studies will never tell you *how* a treatment works or *how* an individual functions, although it may suggest ideas. Neither can any statistical analysis tell anyone exactly how a particular individual, like Karen or you, will respond to a particular treatment. At best it can only provide probabilities. Depending too much on group statistical methods thus promotes a generic approach to activity and exercise.

Such an approach seems well-suited to the mechanized practice of medicine and healthcare that some insurance companies and HMOs have come to encourage. The individuality of each patient can easily get ignored and forgotten in the push to compile statistics and cut costs.

Fortunately, other methods of research are available. If you take the attitude of a personal scientist in regard to your own problem, you don't need to remain completely in the dark about what and what not to do. You can apply the method of possibilities, as discussed in the last chapter, to discover what works for you.

Every person is a unique and different individual. Although similar to others, you are not exactly the same in all respects as anyone else. Therefore, it follows that particular activities and exercises will have their own specific effects on you. By closely observing these effects, it is possible to determine what works best for you. A practitioner who follows such a scientific approach can help you in applying it to your problem and you can learn to do it for yourself (see Chapter 10).

The Problem with 'Posture'

Every type of healthcare practitioner that Karen saw talked with her about her posture. She was consistently told by orthopedists, physical therapists and chiropractors that good posture could help her to restore the proper functioning of her back. She was given written postural instructions as well as stretching and strengthening exercises to improve her posture.

Her experience reflects a significant consensus regarding posture among these different groups.

For example, a brochure on *Low Back Pain* issued by the American Academy of Orthopedic Surgeons states, "The best long-term treatment [for lower back pain] is an active prevention program of maintaining proper lifting and postural activities to prevent further injuries."[24]

The *American Physical Therapy Association Book of Body Maintenance and Repair* states, "Posture has significant implications for the general health and well-being of much of the body...The back, and the lower back in particular, is especially sensitive to proper or poor posture...For your body's sake...it is essential to practice proper posture as much as possible in all activities of daily life."[25]

The American Chiropractic Association issued a policy statement that "...advises and recommends to the public that good posture in all age groups has a direct and significant impact on not only spinal biomechanics but on all bodily functions. Recognition of the interrelationship and interdependence of good posture to good health requires that an increased awareness be developed by the public regarding the necessity of developing good postural habits in order to assist the body in achieving and maintaining good health."[26]

Posture is defined as the relative arrangement of the parts of the body to each other and to the environment. Typically, it is measured, as a person stands, by dropping a plumbline sideways from the tip of the ear to the ankle joint and looking at the alignment of body parts along this vertical line. Alignment is also observed from front and back views of the body.

Good posture (also called "body mechanics" or "use") can be defined as that posture which produces the least strain and maximum efficiency during everyday activities.

This all seems fine and good. But there are hidden quandaries. When people think about 'good posture' they often tend to think of something static and fixed. This is reinforced by how 'posture' is measured, putting a person in a relatively static position or taking a photograph and measuring the alignment of the parts.

It is not that this type of measurement is not useful. It can be. However, the static measurement of posture has been combined with the view of posture as a static and fixed 'thing' and a view of the human organism as a collection of parts to be dealt with separately.

People may then try to impose this static, piecemeal picture on themselves or others by holding themselves in a way that cannot be maintained for long. Or they may try to improve their posture with exercises designed to improve parts of themselves, i.e., range of movement and strength of the back and abdominal muscles, which achieve only partial effects.

This has gone along with a failure to recognize both the general and individual requirements for learning new postural habits. As Karen discovered, the end result has been an emphasis on specific exercises to improve everyday posture. Such exercises are *not sufficient* for changing the moment-to-moment posture that you use in your daily activities. Thus the frustration that many of us have when trying to 'improve' our posture.

"Posture" and "movement" are not necessarily opposites. Even when you seem to be sitting or standing still, there are always some movements going on. The movements of breathing continue, as do the slight swaying or balancing movements that occur when you are standing quietly. Posture always involves movement or activity. Movement or activity always involves some posture.

To acknowledge this relation between posture and movement, some people refer to *static posture* as your posture at rest. This roughly corresponds to sustained positions that we get into. *Dynamic posture* refers to your posture when you move.

I coined the term *"posture-movement"* to make the interrelatedness of posture and movement explicit. Remembering this relation may lead to better posture-movement solutions.

Half-Mast and Full-Sail Self-Care

Most back pain involves activity-related (posture-movement) problems. With less emphasis on bed rest, passive treatments and surgery, we have advanced towards better ways of dealing with these problems. More people understand the general benefits of activity. This has led to more people seeing the importance of self-care and prevention, what the person experiencing back pain can do for herself.

However, just being told to stay active or being given a sheet of generic instructions on exercise and posture is often not enough to take full advantage of the possibilities for self-care. I call this generic approach the 'half-mast' way. A sailboat cannot take advantage of the wind if its sail is not up completely. An approach to prevention cannot work well with cursory, surface efforts.

By contrast, in this book I present a 'full-sail' way of posture-movement self-care. I provide you with the background you need for understanding your back problem and specific principles and methods you can apply to make full use of your potential for self-care.

With my help in applying such methods, Karen no longer feels plagued by chronic pain. Although she has had recurrences, they are less frequent and less severe. Her back moves more easily and she no longer feels the fear that "it is made of glass and will shatter." She is working out at a gym and has begun playing tennis and basketball again for the first time in eight years.

"I was very skeptical when I met you," she wrote to me. "I recall that my first few visits were filtered through my negative thought at the time, 'What is this guy going to do for me?' I've come to realize, it wasn't what *you* did for me. *It's what you taught me to do for myself.*"

Possibilities

Is it possible that the tremendous costs of back pain disability are not inevitable?

Is it possible that the full potential for activity-related methods might be realized by providing a means for comparing theories of what *should* work against the experience of what *actually* does work for individuals?

This book can help you to answer these questions for yourself.

Chapter 3

Back Pain Solutions I: Posture-Movement Therapy

The year was 1981, the place a busy hospital in Pittsburgh. My first glimpse of Paul was of his being wheeled down the hallway of the physical therapy department towards the curtained booth where I would see him. Lying on his back on a gurney, a patient transport table on wheels, he looked nervous.

I felt a little nervous myself, as I often did just before meeting a new patient. I didn't need to feel worried. As a young physical therapist working with people with back pain, I had begun to have a fair amount of success applying the activity-related approaches I had studied.

An New Old Approach to Back Pain

The ancient Chinese and Hindu civilizations both used therapeutic exercise (positions and movements) in their systems of medicine.[1] Posture and movement as therapy also has a long history in the West. More than 2000 years ago, the Greek physician Hippocrates used manipulation and traction to treat people with back pain.[2] Massage and exercise also played important parts in his general practice.[3] In his book *On Articulations* he emphasized the importance of balancing rest with active movement. He wrote:

> ...all parts of the body which have a function, if used in moderation, and exercised in labors to which each is accustomed, become thereby healthy and well-developed, and age slowly; but if unused and left idle, they become liable to disease, defective in growth, and age quickly. This is especially the case with joints and ligaments, if one does not use them. In those who are neglected and never use the leg to walk with but keep it up in the air, the bones are more atrophied than in those who use the leg.[4]

As Erwin H. Ackerknecht noted in his *Short History of Medicine*, Hippocrates also "put great emphasis on the value of observation of the disease process, on the practical rather than the theoretical. This...relegates speculative theories to minor importance."[5]

In later centuries, this activity-related and observation-based approach began to get neglected in relation to back pain. By about 200 years ago, Waddell notes, "restriction of activity, rest and even bed rest [had become] the traditional medical treatment."[6]

Nonetheless, a small number of medical doctors and surgeons, osteopaths, chiropractors and physical therapists, among others, carried on the practice of various forms of activity-related (posture-movement) therapy for back pain with varying degrees of success.

In the twentieth century, James Cyriax, M.D., had a major influence on physical therapists interested in using activity-related therapy for back pain and other musculoskeletal problems. Cyriax promoted a precise method of testing and diagnosing mechanical disorders by observing the effects of postures and movements on symptoms. As he noted, "a change in symptoms corresponding to the stresses acting on the lesion is common to all disorders of the moving parts."[7] He taught simple, precise methods of treatment, particularly manipulation (passive movement), and promoted the use of these methods by physical therapists.

Physical therapists such as Freddy Kaltenborn, Geoffrey Maitland, Stanley Paris and others have carried forward this tradition of activity-related treatment, especially the use of passive movement (manipulative therapy). Maitland, for example, has greatly elaborated on the art of closely observing the relation of the "pain response (its quality and its behavior) to movements and positions."[8] He has taught therapists how to use this pain response as a guide to treatment by means of passive movement.

Physical therapist Robin McKenzie has also advanced activity-related treatment. He and his colleagues emphasize using exercises (movements and static postures carried out by the individual) as a form of self-treatment. As Jacob and McKenzie note, "As with the rehabilitation tradition, the preference is for patient self-generated movements."[9]

In this approach, self-treatment with posture and movement, guided as needed by a therapist, does not preclude the use of passive movements when necessary. However, as self-treatment often works successfully on its own, it seems better to apply it first before going on to manipulative treatment by the therapist. This provides the person with back pain more opportunity to learn how to manage his own symptoms.[10] Paul's story illustrates the usefulness of this approach.

Paul

Paul was a mechanic in his mid-thirties. While he was guiding a heavy engine being put into place with a hoisting device, the chain slipped. Before he had time to think, Paul tried to catch the engine to keep it from falling. He felt something give way in his back. Over a number of weeks the immediate low back pain had gradually spread into his right buttock and down the back of his leg into his calf.

After about two months and despite some physical therapy and chiropractic treatments, the pain was now constant and disturbing his sleep. Sitting and bending were agony, as were standing and walking any distance. He was unable to work. He had been admitted to the hospital for a workup, including a myelogram, prior to anticipated surgery for a herniated disc.

A myelogram is a special x-ray test wherein fluid is first injected into the spinal canal. This fluid makes it possible to see dents in the lower spinal cord and nerves which can indicate if and in what location a herniated disc may be pressing on nerve tissue. Paul's myelogram was scheduled for the next day.

Paul was in the clinic this day for some 'palliative' treatment: heat, ultrasound, massage and flexion exercise. I got a history of his problem from him and carefully (he was in constant, severe pain) tested the reflexes, sensation and muscle strength in his legs. Although he had pain and tingling in his right calf, the results seemed normal.

To comply with the orthopedist's orders to do flexion exercises, I asked Paul to pull his knees to his chest. Paul was willing to try. However, the pain in his calf increased and spread into his foot after only a few movements. I decided that flexion exercises were *not* for him right now. I asked him to stop and roll over onto his stomach (a static prone-lying posture). He moved slowly and carefully, in evident pain, and I went to get the heat pack.

Knowing how positions and movements can affect symptoms, when I returned I asked him how far the pain in his right leg extended. His foot had stopped hurting and tingling—however, he felt intense discomfort going down to his mid-calf.

I helped him to lift himself up while I placed a pillow under his belly to see if this might make a difference. He felt no worse. I helped him lift up again to place another pillow. This time the pain retreated up to the back of his knee. I was encouraged because the site of his pain had changed by changing his position. I placed the hotpack on his back and left the room for a few minutes.

When I returned, Paul reported that his knee felt better. He felt pain from his back and buttock down to his mid-thigh, a good sign. The pain was "centralizing," a term McKenzie uses to describe symptoms moving out of the limb and towards the spine (see the section on Soft Tissue Changes in Chapter 9). So I left Paul with both pillows and the hot pack, which was basically there to distract him and keep him still.

After five minutes his symptoms had not significantly changed. I decided to see what would happen if I removed first one pillow and then the second. After he settled back down on the table, with his spine in a basically neutral position, he reported no pain in his thigh, only in his back and buttock.

An hour later, my supervisor was wondering why I was keeping my patient so long and Paul was doing press-ups, an exercise during which he repeatedly extended his spine —bent it backwards—by pushing up with his arms while lying on his stomach (Exercise #3 in Chapter 10). He had some difficulty doing this. The movement was limited. However, the pain in his leg and butt had vanished. Although the right-sided back pain was still present, it had shifted closer to the center of his back. It had taken more than an hour, with many gradual adjustments of pillows and body position on the table, but both Paul and I felt elated.

Paul's orthopedic surgeon had his office next to the physical therapy clinic. I ran over to talk with him. I described what I had done with Paul and how he had responded. I requested that the order be changed to extension exercises and explained my rationale for doing so. At the time, flexion exercises were prescribed almost universally in the U.S. and this approach, using extension when appropriate, was not well known or accepted. He looked skeptical but agreed and I beat a hasty retreat.

Back in the clinic, Paul's arms felt sore. He had done 40 press-ups while waiting for me to return. But although he felt moderate pain across his lower back, he felt much better overall, with no buttock or leg pain. I suggested he do the exercises every couple of hours, and sent him back to his room.

Paul returned to the clinic the next morning. He had a small amount of constant back pain which, with exercise and a brief use of passive movement (spinal manipulation) applied by me, he was able to get rid of by the afternoon's session. His myelogram had been cancelled. He was discharged the following day and continued coming for about 3 weeks as an outpatient, until he had returned to full duty at work and was entirely pain-free. On his last visit he thanked me for helping him to avoid surgery.

Posture-Movement Therapy

As Paul discovered, the effectiveness for an individual of activity-related treatment does not depend on abstract theories or statistics. Neither a theory nor a statistic will indicate exactly how you as an individual will respond to a treatment. Rather, treating you as an individual requires an empirical, observational approach.

Taking the attitude of a personal scientist, you can determine what works for you. Applying some of the insights of Hippocrates, Cyriax, Maitland and others, you can become a better observer as you explore the possibilities of posture and movement to reduce your pain and improve your functioning. In this way, you can become a better consumer of the healthcare services that you receive. Using the insights of McKenzie, you especially can explore the role of self-treatment in posture-movement therapy. (Chapter 10 details a set of positions and movements that you may find useful.)

What positions and movements reduce your symptoms and improve your ability to move?

This chapter has introduced you to some of the background and application of posture-movement therapy. This approach to therapy solutions for back pain works together with educational solutions which I explore in the next chapter.

Chapter 4

Back Pain Solutions II:
Posture-Movement Education

The Problem of Habit

As I saw more and more people with back and neck problems, I continued to have many successes. I found that people often were able to control their symptoms through exercises using different positions and movements, with manipulative treatment (passive movements) supplementing this when needed. As part of this work, I also emphasized the importance of dynamic posture in daily life. However, as the following story shows, I discovered difficulties in helping people adopt new, healthier habits.

One day, while visiting a friend's house, I noticed something different about his 15-year-old son. I had gotten used to seeing Jeremy slumping, his spine in the shape of a big letter C and his head protruding in front of the rest of his body. This day, although this usual posture hadn't changed, Jeremy moved carefully and stiffly. What was the problem?

Jeremy had woken up with a pain in his neck and upper back on one side. He had difficulty turning his head. He had no idea what had caused this to happen all of a sudden. I asked him and his father if I could help. Knowing that I worked as a physical therapist who specialized in this kind of problem, they both agreed.

I first asked Jeremy to tell me a little bit about the pain. (See Index Your Symptoms, in Chapter 10, for more on the skill of accurately describing symptoms.) Jeremy's pain felt constant. That is, he noticed some discomfort even when resting. I asked him to show me on his body exactly where he felt the pain. It spread from the right side of his neck and upper back to several inches along the top of his right shoulder blade.

His head and neck movements appeared restricted and painful, especially towards the right. He also couldn't extend his head and neck very far back to look up towards the ceiling.

I asked him to rate his symptoms on a scale from 0 to 10, with 0 meaning no pain and 10 meaning the worst that he could imagine. Using a simple scale like this provides a way to become a better observer of your symptoms and thus to practice being a personal scientist. Jeremy said it felt like a 6.

I explained to him that these kinds of symptoms are often related to positions and movements of the body. Seeing his greatly distorted protruded-head position, I thought that working on his posture would be a good place to start.

I asked him if he would allow me to help him to experience a different position of his head and neck in order to see what effect it would have on his symptoms. He agreed to this and I invited him to sit on a chair. I proceeded very gently to guide him into a position where his back was no longer rounded and his neck and head were brought back closer to the top of his spine. This took several minutes, during which time I talked with him, asking him to let go of tensions or holding here and there and encouraging him to let me know how he was feeling.

After getting repositioned, he sat erect, an unusual position to see him in. He himself felt quite odd, almost crooked. I asked him what he felt in his neck. There was now only a small amount of discomfort, about a 3, along his spine in the mid to lower neck. Just changing his sitting posture had changed his symptoms for the better. Interestingly enough, his ability to move had also improved. With my hands gently guiding his head and neck movements, he could now turn his neck more fully to both sides with little increase in pain.

Since I had to leave soon, I reviewed the importance of everyday posture in the best way that I could under the circumstances. I demonstrated good and bad postures and explained how maintaining good posture would help. He acknowledged that he already had experienced evidence of this.

Then I instructed him in the "chin-tuck" exercise (described in Chapter 15), a movement that emphasizes the opposite direction of his habitual protruded-head position. He had some difficulty doing it on his own and I guided him through the movement with my hands. The small amount of pain decreased and, after about twenty repetitions, had altogether vanished.

While I talked with his father, Jeremy walked around for a few minutes. After awhile I could see that he had begun to return to his habitual slump. When I asked he said that some of the neck pain, not as severe, had also returned. I urged him to do the exercise I showed him, even if he had a bit of trouble with doing it correctly.

I didn't see him again until several weeks later. He was slumping as much as ever. When I asked him how he was doing, he thanked me. He had done the exercises and corrected his posture as best he could and he reported that he had no pain. Given his slumping, how long-lasting would this be, I wondered.

Working with people with back, neck and other activity-related pain, I had many similar experiences. A few people, who it clearly seemed could benefit from improving their posture, didn't see the point. "I've slumped all my life," they might say, "but I just started having pain in my back so how can you tell me that my posture is a problem?"

Many others did see the point but despite their best efforts to comply often were unable to maintain the good postures that I showed them for sitting, bending and moving. And more often than not, people thought they were doing the exercises correctly and moving with better posture and body mechanics when they weren't.

It seemed clear here that so-called 'subjective' or 'mental' factors—people's desire to change, their body awareness, their willingness to experience themselves in new and unfamiliar ways and their persistence and willingness to work, among other factors—had as much importance as the 'objective' exercises and instructions I gave them.

Fortunately, what people *could* do often seemed good enough temporarily. But I felt frustrated about not being able to make further inroads in helping people change their habits —habits that might prolong their symptoms and make them more vulnerable to future episodes of pain. I wondered about the bent-over elderly people I saw in the hospitals and nursing facilities where I had worked, as well as on the street. To what extent was this condition due to years of postural neglect?

My study of therapy approaches had brought me to the edge of what appeared to be an educational problem. It is easy to treat your body as an object and let your attention go somewhere else while doing exercises. This can reinforce the illusion that there is a separate 'mind' and separate 'body'. Then you can neglect the so-called 'mental' aspect. However, for posture-movement education to have any chance of success, 'subjective', or 'mental' factors, cannot be left out.

Education and 'Body'–'Mind' Unity

By the time I went to physical therapy school in the late 70s and early 80s, lip service—perhaps more commonly given nowadays—was already being paid to the unity of the 'mind and the 'body' (ironically, by talking in terms of two separate things—the 'mind' and the 'body').

In practice the split of 'body' and 'mind' pervaded physical therapy and medicine, as it does today. The approaches I learned in physical therapy school emphasized the 'body' as a machine made of isolated parts and downplayed or neglected the role of the inner life (consciousness) of the individual.

Understanding the mechanisms (how they work) of nerves, muscles, joints, exercise, etc., was and still is considered 'objective' and 'scientific'. Understanding the role of consciousness—the mechanisms (how they work) of my own inner life and that of the individuals I sought to help—was considered 'subjective' and less 'scientific', or at least not a part of 'real science'.

As a physical therapy student, I observed that the best clinicians and teachers were able to unify the so-called 'objective' and 'subjective' elements in their work. Nonetheless, my interest in dealing with both the outer and inner person seemed odd and peripheral to the main business of exercise science that I studied.

As a student of the practical philosophy of General Semantics, I had already rejected the divisions of 'objective' and 'subjective', 'body' and 'mind', as unsound.

With biologist C.H. Waddington, I agreed that:

> An attempt to make a clean cut break between the subjective mental observer and the objective material observed [what philosopher Alfred North Whitehead called the 'Bifurcation of Nature'], is a basic error. They are initially parts of a whole, and if one wants for some purposes to separate them, that can only be a matter of convenience that should be indulged in with great caution.[1]

I began to put this understanding into practice by becoming more aware of my language and that of others. I worked to remember what general semanticist Alfred Korzybski wrote:

> Linguistic and grammatical structure also have prevented our study of human reactions. For instance, we used and still use a terminology of 'objective' and 'subjective', both extremely confusing, as the so-called 'objective' must be

considered a construct made by our nervous system, and what we call 'subjective' may also be considered 'objective' for the same reasons.[2]

I began to think, talk and write about myself and others in terms of Korzybski's phrase "organisms-as-wholes-in-environments."[3] I worked at remembering that successfully dealing with the living reactions of individuals (myself included) must involve the so-called 'subjective' factors as nervous system functions of the organism. I began exploring practical methods of working with people that did not divide a fictional 'mind' from a fictional 'body'. These studies included Sensory Awareness (discussed in Chapter 12) and F.M. Alexander's work. Eventually I became a teacher of the Alexander Technique.

A New Old Approach to Posture-Movement Education

Posture-movement education almost undoubtedly goes back to the first efforts of early humans to help their young learn the motor skills related to hunting, gathering and other aspects of daily life. Written records of posture-movement education can be found in accounts of the several-thousand-year-old practices of Chinese Kung-Fu (Qigong), Indian Yoga and Greek and Roman gymnastics, which paralleled the work in therapy that I discussed in the last chapter.[4]

In Europe in recent centuries, singing teachers and voice coaches focused on their students' posture habits in relation to breathing and movement.[5]

During this same period, posture-movement education also continued in the work of a number of physicians and associated workers in physical education. These people realized the importance of engaging the body-mind (organism-as-a-whole-in-an-environment) when working to help people with posture, movement and breathing difficulties.[6]

Probably influenced by translations of Chinese Qigong texts,[7] the Swedish Gymnastics movement founded by Pehr

Ling, had particular importance in both the medical and non-medical areas.[8,9]

Dr. Mathias Roth wrote this about Ling's system of Medical Gymnastics in his 1856 *Handbook of the Movement Cure*:

> The oneness of the human organism, and the harmony between mind and body, and between the various parts of the same body, constitute the great principle of Ling's gymnastics.

> The development and preservation of the harmony between mind and body, as well as among the various organs of the body, is the object of Ling's system with regard to healthy persons, and this is the educational or prophylactic part of the system, while the restoration of the disturbed harmony of the different organs produced by diseases, forms the object of the medical part.[10]

It is against this background that Australian-English actor F. Matthias Alexander (1869–1955) sought a solution to the vocal problems that he developed in the last decade of the nineteenth century.

According to Alexander's account in his 1932 book, *The Use of the Self*,[11] he worked over a period of time observing himself in the act of speaking. Although obscure about his sources, it seems likely that in order to work out his own problems he supplemented his self-observations with study of some of the available literature and consultation with professionals in the field.[12]

"Synthesizing parts from voice pedagogy and physical therapy," as Ed Bouchard and Ben Wright state in their book *Kinesthetic Ventures,* Alexander "...developed a 'technique' employing gentle touch to teach natural posture and breathing essential to effective vocal use."[13] This work has also been found effective in working with people with back pain and other posture-movement related problems.

Alexander's synthesis follows a number of basic principles. Patrick Macdonald, a student of Alexander's who became a well-known teacher of his technique, listed these as follows (modified by me and in a different order):

Recognition of the Force of Habit
Head-Neck-Back Relations
Importance of Sensation/Perception
Inhibition
Sending Directions [14]

I will briefly discuss each of these notions in turn, as together they cover some of the main issues of posture-movement education.

Recognition of the Force of Habit

Alexander emphasized the role habit plays in our posture and movement. William James, in his 1890 classic *Principles of Psychology,* had already written a great deal about habits. In a lecture based on this work he said:

All our life, so far as it has definite form, is but a mass of habits, — practical, emotional, and intellectual, — systematically organized for our weal or woe, and bearing us irresistibly toward our destiny, whatever the latter may be.[15]

James wrote directly about posture-movement habits (what Alexander called "the use of the self") in his essay, "The Gospel of Relaxation":

The general over-contraction may be small when estimated in foot-pounds, but its importance is immense on account of its *effects on the over-contracted person's spiritual life.* ...For by the sensations that so incessantly pour in from the over-tense excited body the over-tense and excited habit of mind is kept up.... [O]ver-tension and jerkiness are primarily social, and only secondarily physiological, phenomena. They are *bad habits*, nothing more or less, bred of the imitation of bad models and the cultivation of false personal ideals.[16]

As Alexander found, those who seek to help themselves or others move towards better posture will need to deal in one way or another with the force of habit.

Head-Neck-Back Relations

In his later writings, Alexander emphasized the importance of the relations among the head and neck, the back and the rest of the body. Years after his initial explorations, he noted that these relations constituted "the primary control" for body use (posture-movement habits).[17]

Talking about "*the* primary control" can imply that something exists as a more-or-less separate and all important entity. Some have attempted to locate "the primary control" in a single part of the anatomy or as an isolated physiological function. However, the mutual, dynamic postural relations among the head, neck, back (spine), torso and limbs exist in a larger context of the external environment, a person's internal physiology and his/her conscious state. These complex interrelations make it inadvisable to label any one part or factor 'the primary control'.

Nonetheless, in posture-movement education, the head, neck and back (spine) relations do have importance. Many recognized this prior to Alexander.

Japanese, Chinese and Indian practitioners in various meditative and movement practices recognized long ago the importance of the head, neck and back in "right posture."[18]

The singing teachers and teachers of medical gymnastics mentioned before taught this as well. Scanes Spicer, M.D., a physician who studied these approaches and with whom Alexander was acquainted, wrote early in this century about the importance of the head, neck and spine in posture education for respiratory and other problems.[19]

These students of posture and movement understood the mutual relations among the limbs, the lower torso (the belly and lower back), the rest of the torso (chest and upper back) and the neck and head. They knew that inadequate support from below can encourage poor posture of the head and neck. In turn, habitually tightening the neck and pulling the head backwards, or letting it slump into this position, can encourage a downward direction and shortening of the rest of the body. This is the protruded head position that Jeremy habitually assumed.

By contrast, adequate support from below allows freedom in the neck so that the head can move from the backwards-pulled position to a more forward and upright one. This means, in Spicer's words, a "passive, loose balance of head on spine; no active muscular tension or rigidity."[20] In turn, this encourages a continuing upward direction and lengthening of the rest of the body with "fullest spinal extension...straightening out not only dorsal spine (to enlarge chest), but also cervical spine (to enlarge throat) and lumbar spine (to make room for viscera backwards)."[21] This is the more neutral, erect position that Jeremy assumed with my help. Figure 4.1 illustrates the head and neck portion of these two contrasting postures.

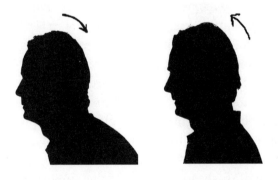

Figure 4.1 – Head Back and Down vs. Forward and Up

A phrase used by Alexander summarizes this second, more beneficial posture: "Let the neck be free, to let the head go forward and up, to let the back lengthen and widen."

Importance of Sensation/Perception

Our sensations/perceptions play a major role in our posture-movement habits. Observing himself and others, Alexander noted what his student Macdonald called "faulty sensory awareness." We may not have an adequate sense of what we are doing with ourselves. Someone who mistakenly perceives himself as already having good static and dynamic posture will not see the need to correct it.

Before and since the time that Alexander presented his system, others working in the field of posture-movement education have been aware of the fallibility of our senses and the importance of improving awareness in relation to our posture and movement.

Dr. Mathias Roth, whose work influenced Spicer (and quite likely Alexander as well), published *An Essay on the Prevention and Rational Treatment of Lateral Spinal Curvature* in 1885. Roth noted:

> The majority of patients suffering from various forms of spinal curvatures are not aware of their abnormal position; they feel straight while in a crooked position, and while the spine is curved; the spinal curvature is usually accompanied by compensating abnormal position of the head.[22]

Roth advises that with training, sensation can become a more reliable guide to posture and movement:

> The majority of patients being unconscious of their abnormal position, the first object to be obtained is to change the false mental impression they have in believing themselves straight when they are crooked, and feeling crooked when placed in a normal position. The second object is to enable the patients to retain the normal position, which at first causes the sensation of being crooked.[23]

In keeping with this, Alexander worked at developing hands-on teaching methods to help students gain more trustworthy sensations/perceptions related to better body use. As he said:

Surely...if it is possible for feeling to become untrustworthy as a means of direction, it should also be possible to make it trustworthy again. [24]

Inhibition

In *The Use of the Self,* Alexander described how he gradually became more conscious of the abnormal positions and movements ruining his voice. He also gradually began to change the false impression he had of his posture and movement and to experience better, more normal positions.

However, once he had begun to realize a better way of using himself while speaking, he found that he couldn't retain it. He still often continued with his old, bad posture-movement habits.

These included pulling his head back and downwards on his neck. At the same time he would compress and tighten his throat, puff out his chest and ribs, arch his back and tighten his legs and grip his feet on the floor, among other things. He could see and feel that this excessive effort interfered with his breathing even as it involved greater and greater pushing to get his voice out.

Observing the effects of faulty sensory awareness in himself, he also saw that his problem was not simply 'physical'. It started with his intention to speak. As soon as he formulated the idea of speaking he could observe himself tightening his neck, pulling his head back and down, and initiating the rest of his pattern of excessive tension.

Alexander experimented with pausing before he actually spoke. While he did this, he consciously focused on not going into the old pattern. This idea of pausing, or stopping and not doing some intended action, had been applied by others[25] and became an important aspect of what Alexander taught. He called it "inhibition," a term used in various works of psychology available at the time. Alexander combined inhibition, or delaying the immediate response to a situation, with what he called the process of "sending directions."

Sending Directions

While Alexander observed himself with mirrors—as recommended in the physical therapy of the time[26]—he practiced sending "directions" or "orders." These were subvocal instructions that he gave to himself, which included negative directions. He thus reminded himself to delay his response to speak and to not pull his head back, etc.

Alexander's negative directions qualified as, in William James' words, "inhibition by repression or negation." James had pointed out the danger of focusing too much on what not to do where "both the inhibited ideal and the inhibiting ideal...remain along with each other in consciousness, producing a certain inward strain or tension there."[27]

Alexander wisely sought to reduce this strain by also sending positive directions—positive subvocal verbal instructions for proper use that he gave himself. The words served as aids for him to direct his attention to himself: "Let the neck be free, to let the head go forward and up, to let the back lengthen and widen."

This second, positive use of directions allowed him to practice what James called "inhibition by substitution," wherein "the inhibiting idea supersedes altogether the idea which it inhibits, and the latter quickly vanishes from the field."[28] The positive instructions for good use helped him substitute for, and supersede, the poor use. This positive use of directions may have greater usefulness than the negative. James noted:

> It is clear that in general we ought, whenever we can, to employ the method of inhibition by substitution....Spinoza long ago wrote in his *Ethics* that anything a man can avoid under the notion that it is bad he may also avoid under the notion that something else is good.[29]

Continuing to observe himself in the mirror, Alexander could confirm that he was not doing what he didn't want to do. He could also see that he was doing what he wanted to do. His sensory awareness became more reliable. With practice he found that he could continue his good body use while speaking and with other activities of daily living as well. He could thus avoid the habitual strain to which he previously had been accustomed.

James had written "*To think*...is the secret of will...."[30] Whether Alexander read William James' work directly is unknown. But the ideas of the new psychology, research in hypnosis, as well as popular watered-down versions of this work involving so-called mind cures, etc., were in the air. Earlier medical practitioners like Roth had emphasized the importance of sensory awareness and the conscious direction of will to deal with posture-movement problems. Again, more ancient practitioners had gotten there first. The Chinese Qigong classics advised: "Use intent, not force."[31]

Did Alexander re-discover this completely on his own? Who knows? Nonetheless, it is a powerful notion which he used and taught to others. Posture-movement habits can best be improved not with stretching or strengthening exercises (force) but with the 'exercise' of thought and awareness (directed intent) in daily life.

Alexander's Contribution

In seeking to solve his own vocal problems, Alexander brought together the notions of direction, inhibition and the other elements discussed previously into a unique system of posture-movement education.

A strong sense of ethical concern permeates his approach —characterized by the realization that ends and means exist inseparably from one another. In connection with your everyday posture-movement habits, if you use stress-inducing body mechanics as your means, the ends you actually achieve will more likely include pain and inefficiency. Aldous Huxley, who took lessons from Alexander, pointed out that this can serve as a exemplar for the larger area of human ethical action.[32]

Alexander's contribution to posture-movement education has been well-summarized by posture-movement researcher and Alexander Technique teacher Ron Dennis:

> In what must now appear as a variously-sourced synthesis, Alexander's creative contribution needs clear acknowledgment. If he did not, on the one hand, singlehandedly reveal an entire new field of endeavor, he did, on the other, succeed in fashioning, from heretofore disparate elements, a distinctively harmonious system, one praised by contemporary physicians as 'a very advanced craft and a very subtle philosophy',* and one moreover imbued with an ethos of self-help not merely for symptomatic relief but for the very rightness of it all. This ethical aspect of 'the Work' may well have been what drew such eminent thinkers as John Dewey, Aldous Huxley and George Bernard Shaw, as well as numerous others, to it. [33]
>
> [*The reference is from *The Use of the Self*, Appendix, Letter of May 8, 1930, from Drs. Cameron, Douglas, et al.]

The Skill of Everyday Living

A. N. Whitehead wrote that "Familiar things happen, and mankind does not bother about them. It requires a very unusual mind to undertake the analysis of the obvious."[34] We easily recognize the skill involved in the feats of Olympic and professional athletes. Yet most of us do not recognize the complexity of skill involved in the the most obvious activities of everyday living.

C.S. Sherrington, an 'unusual mind' who helped found modern neuroscience, once observed:

> [Standing] requires among other things the right degree of action of a great many muscles and nerves, some thousands of nerve-fibres and of perhaps a hundred times as many muscle-fibres. In doing so my brain's rightness of action rests on receiving and adjusting pressures, tensions etc. in various parts of me.[35]

Our everyday skilled acts may involve unnecessary effort that can have cumulative harmful effects on how we function. This can contribute to back pain, among other problems. Sherrington also observed:

> Breathing, standing, walking, sitting, although innate, along with our growth, are apt as movements, to suffer from defects in our ways of doing them. A chair unsuited to a child can quickly induce special and bad habits of sitting, and of breathing. In urbanized and industrialized communities bad habits in our motor acts are especially common.[36]

Perhaps because we do not usually think of our basic acts as skills, we do not take advantage of the possibilities for improving them. Dennis has emphasized that posture-movement education, as exemplified by the Alexander Technique, focuses on helping you acquire greater skill in your mostly unconsciously acquired activities of daily living.[37] In developing your posture-movement skills, you can reduce the stress on your back and other parts and improve your level of efficiency and comfort.

Posture-movement therapy, discussed in the previous chapter, focuses on using particular postures and movements to alleviate specific symptoms. It provides an "exercise" approach for dealing with your back problems.

Posture-movement education, because it focuses on awareness and intent in your everyday activities, provides an "un-exercise" approach—as Dennis has called it—to enhance your posture-movement skills.[38]

In Part II (the next three chapters) you will learn how your back is constructed. You will find out what happens when you experience pain. You will read about principles of learning applicable to controlling your pain and your body use. These chapters may seem a bit theoretical and you may be tempted to skip them to get to "the good parts." Of course, you can do so if you wish and still benefit from what you read. However,

I suggest that, if you read these chapters first, you will have more of the necessary background for understanding the "exercise" approach of Part III and the "un-exercise" approach of Part IV, which follow.

Part II
Necessary Background

> Knowledge: A little light expels much darkness.
> - Bahya Ibn Paquda[1]

Chapter 5

How Your Back Works

Your beliefs play a large part in helping or not helping you to get what you want. How do you evaluate your back pain? Do you think that your pain represents punishment for your 'sins'? Or perhaps you think that it's a mysterious thing that just happens and that you have no control over it? These beliefs will surely lead to different results than if you think you have an activity-related problem possibly correctable through posture and movement.

I want to help you to evaluate your back problem more effectively. In order to do this, I will use the next three chapters to present certain background information that you can use to understand your problem. In this chapter, I provide basic information on the anatomy and physiology of your back. Chapter 6 discusses pain, how it works and how your system is built to deal with it. Then Chapter 7 presents a basic outline of Perceptual Control Theory (PCT), a theory of human behavior based on feedback principles, that provides a conceptual framework for learning how to control your pain and your posture-movement habits.

Them Bones, Them Joints, Them Muscles, Them Nerves

It's been said that your spine is a column. You sit on one end and your head sits on the other.[1] Be that as it may, in order to take care of your back, you may find it useful to know more than "the back bone's connected to the head bone." If you find yourself becoming intimidated by unfamiliar medical terms, just read on. You don't need to understand everything in order to begin to feel a bit more comfortable and familiar with the parts and functions of your body.

Before discussing the specific parts of the back, I'll briefly review the different types of structures involved in our sensing-moving system, that is, the *Neuro-Musculo-Skeletal* (NMS) system. *Neuro* here refers to the nervous system: the brain, spinal cord and nerves that go to and from every part of the body. *Musculo* refers to the muscles that create movement and that make up approximately 40% of the weight of the human body. *Skeletal* refers to the bones and joints.

Let's look at the *Skeletal* aspect first. The *bones* provide the framework of the body and the actual segments that move. We may think of them as solid and unchanging but the bones are anything but inert, since they can change shape according to the mechanical forces, like muscle pulls, that work on them.

A joint is a place where bones meet (see Figure 5.1). Movement occurs (for the most part) where joints are located. The majority of joints are *synovial joints* and consist of the adjoining ends of the respective bones and a surrounding envelope of *connective tissue* called the *joint capsule*. The shapes at the ends of the bones determine the direction of movement that occurs at the joint. The ends of the bones are covered by *cartilage*, which is the firm but spongy white covering that you see at the ends of chicken bones sometimes.

The cartilage secretes a fluid that fills the joint capsule and lubricates between the cartilage surfaces of the bones, allowing for smooth movements. The outside of the capsule is reinforced with *ligaments*, which are tough connective tissue structures attached to the adjoining bones. Ligaments limit excessive or abnormal movement.

Now let's look at the *Musculo* part of the NMS system. Muscles typically are attached across a joint from one bone to another. They are attached to the bones by means of *tendons*, which are also formed from connective tissue. The bones, cartilage, joint capsules, ligaments and tendons can all be considered *passive tissues* because they do not move by themselves. Muscles can be considered the *active tissues* of the NMS system because, when signaled by nerve impulses, they can actively create tension, contract, and change their length.

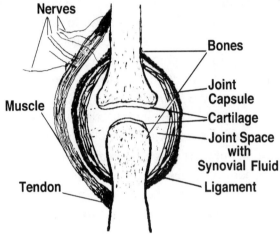

Figure 5.1 – Joint-Muscle Complex

This leaves us with the last, *Neuro,* aspect of the NMS system to consider. *Spinal nerves* exit from the spinal cord and bind into "cables" called *peripheral nerves.* These course through the torso and limbs. Since the individual nerve fibers are bound together by connective tissue sheaths, they are capable of getting stretched, compressed and sometimes injured by mechanical forces. Impulses carried in the nerves signal the muscles to contract. The nerves also provide the sensory connections from muscles, tendons, joints, skin, etc., which provide input to the *Central Nervous System (CNS).*

The CNS consists of the brain, encased in the skull, and the spinal cord, which is housed within the central opening of the spine, called the spinal canal. The CNS provides the main control system for the organism. The brain and spinal cord are surrounded by connective tissue sheaths, which are continuous with those surrounding the peripheral nerves. The nervous system is illustrated in Figure 5.2.

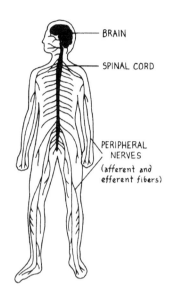

Figure 5.2 – Nervous System

The nerves to the muscles (efferent fibers) are the final common pathways of signals from the CNS. Messages from sensors in the muscles as well as the tendons, ligaments and joints also travel back into the CNS control areas (afferent fibers). This feedback, some of which we can become conscious of, is important. To the extent that we can perceive various aspects of our posture and movement, we have the potential to control them.

The Movement Chain

Like the rest of the organism, the NMS system works as a whole. Whether you write your name in the sand with your finger or your toe or turn off the light switch with your elbow or your nose, it's not just the toe or the nose that's involved. No part of the moving system works in isolation.

Rather, the movement of finger or elbow is the end point of a *movement (kinematic) chain*[2]—a linkage of body segments connected through the joints that goes from the tips of the toes to the neck and head. A seemingly insignificant movement of one part of the body requires muscular and joint adjustments, however slight, in other parts. What happens at one end of this movement chain can impact what happens at the other end.

You can experience this kind of 'chain reaction' by sitting slumped, with your back in a collapsed C curve. Stay in this position while you try to raise your arms over your head. Notice how far your arms go. Now consciously sit erect. (For the purposes of this demonstration, it doesn't matter if this is a little forced). Again raise your arms and notice how far you can bring them over your head. Did you find that you could raise your arms further when sitting erect? This illustrates how the configuration of one part of the chain can affect movement of another part.

Professional athletes are sometimes more aware than the rest of us of these chainlike connections. Picture a baseball pitcher winding up at the mound. A pitcher throws not just with his arm but with his whole body (functions as an organism-as a-whole-in-an-environment).

Martial arts experts also emphasize this kind of whole body relationship. Tai Chi Grand Master William C. C. Chen has talked about how "If you are loose and the body is coordinated you will have power using the whole body. The whole body moving as a unit. That is my whole concept." [3]

Just keeping awareness that your whole body can be involved in a movement can keep you from unduly isolating a part like your back. It's important to realize that your back has 'friends' and 'neighbors' within the movement chain. The different parts can function together so that less stress is taken by any part. Looking at a skeleton can help you to see some of these bodily connections. If you don't have access to an actual skeleton (other than your own) or a plastic model, a picture will do for now. See Figure 5.3.

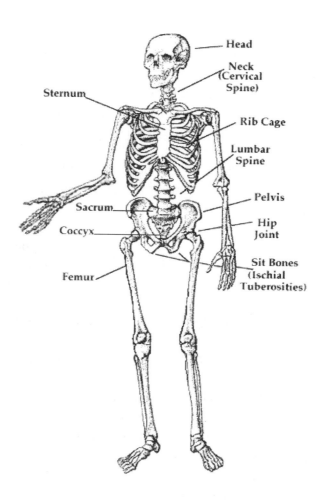

Figure 5.3 — Human Skeleton

A Personal Anatomy Tour

The head, spine, rib cage and pelvis represent the central framework of your body. Together they form the core, or axis, of your body's framework.

The upper and lower limbs make up the appendages to this central framework.

Let's locate the different parts of your skeleton in order to define them more clearly (not just with other words but with experiences).

Feel your head with your hands. Your head, as I said, sits at one end of your spine. Do you know where that sitting place is actually located? If you place each index finger in the hollow just behind your earlobes, your fingers will be pointing approximately at the level at which your head sits on top of your first *cervical* (neck) bone or vertebra (medical-speak for spinal bone). The first cervical is also called the *"atlas,"* in honor of the Titan of Greek mythology who held up the world.

With your fingers still in place, delicately nod your head in a "yes" motion. Two rounded knobs at the bottom of the skull sit on top of two concave hollows on the atlas and allow that slight rocking motion to take place.

The atlas, in turn, sits like a ring positioned over the protruding posterior 'finger' of the second cervical vertebra, the *axis*. This arrangement facilitates your head rotating on your neck.

Seven neck bones are stacked one on top of the other. Feel around the back of your neck and move your fingers down the midline until you come to a bump. That bump is probably the palpable back portion of the seventh and last cervical bone.

So the cervical or neck portion of your spine extends from the base of your skull (level with where you previously placed your fingers) to the level of that bump, the seventh cervical vertebra.

The neck region as a whole includes all of the structures (muscles, nerves, glands, throat, etc.) within the length that the bones define. The joints of your neck allow a great deal of flexibility for flexing, extending, side-bending and rotation movements.

The twelve *thoracic* vertebrae link up the next portion of your spine. These bones link with the *ribs*, which are connected in front to the *sternum* or *breastbone*. The area encircled within the ribs, thoracic vertebrae and sternum contains the lungs and other vital organs. Your ribs are able to move, which allows for the expansion and contraction of your lungs.

Gently press the palms of your hands along the front of your rib cage just above the navel. Can you feel the movement there as you breathe? The thoracic vertebrae themselves have less movement than that of the neck, due to the rib attachments and the shape of the bones. They have some flexion (forward bending) and rotation ability as well as sidebending, with a very limited amount of extension (backward bending).

The five lower back or *lumbar* vertebrae are thicker than the ones above. They are approximately at belt level. These bones can sometimes be felt, especially when lying flat or bending forwards. The lumbar vertebrae have significant amounts of flexion and extension, with lesser amounts of side bending and rotation.

The lowest portions of the spine, the *sacrum* and *coccyx (tailbone)*, consist of fused spinal bones that are wedged like an inverted triangle at the rear of the *pelvis* between the bones of the pelvis. The fibrous, immovable joint between the sacrum and pelvic bone (the ilium) on either side is called the *sacroiliac joint* and is reinforced by a number of strong ligament connections between the bones.

As you look at a standing side view of the whole length of the spine in Figure 5.4, you can see its characteristic four curves. In the normal adult spine, the cervical spine usually appears concave (hollowed) towards the back. The thoracic part of the spine curves convexly (bump outwards) towards the back. The lumbar spine again has a concavity or hollow called the *lumbar lordosis*. Finally, the fused sacrum and coccyx are curved convexly (bump outwards) towards the back.

These curves are gradually formed from infancy as we develop our upright posture. Our tendency to form them results from the evolutionary adaptation to standing erect, which was made 4 or 5 million years ago by our smaller-brained, but upright and walking predecessors.

This adaptation can be explained by the engineering discovery that the resistance to compression of a column increases if it is curved. Consider just the three curves above the sacrum: the cervical, thoracic and lumbar portion of the spinal column has 10 times more resistance to compression than it would if it were entirely straight.[4]

Some people claim that the prevalence of back pain has something to do with an imperfect human adaptation to the vertical position. However, the presence of these curves shows that some evolutionary adaptation has occurred. Reversing evolution by returning to walking on all four limbs (except occasionally) does not seem practical.

Your habits and life style can lead you to spend too much time with one or more of your spinal curves either reduced or exaggerated. In this way, you can lessen your spine's resistance to mechanical stress. You can benefit by looking at how you can change these habits.

Continuing your anatomy tour to your pelvis, feel the bony shelves on either side of your 'waist'. These are often called the 'hip bones' and confused with the hip joints, which I will discuss below. What you feel are the top edges or 'wings' of the pelvis. They are at about the level of the fourth and fifth lumbar vertebrae.

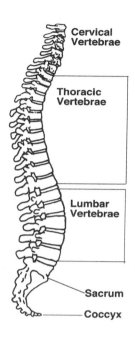

Cervical
Vertebrae

Thoracic
Vertebrae

Lumbar
Vertebrae

Sacrum

Coccyx

Figure 5.4 — The Spinal Curves

The pelvis itself consists of a combination of three paired bones. The two large bony knobs on each side that make contact with the chair when you're sitting are the sit bones (*ischial tuberosities*) of the pelvis.

On either side, the pelvis forms the the socket portion of the ball-and-socket hip joint. The ball part is at the top of the thighbone (*femur*). The hip joint is too deep to be felt directly but is located inside the crease of the groin which bends when you flex your upper leg or when you bend forwards when sitting or standing.

Together, the pelvis, spine and ribs, with all that they contain, comprise the *torso*. The upper and lower back region is simply the back part of the torso. This completes our tour of the central framework of your body—your torso, neck and head.

If you haven't done so, I suggest that you find these different parts on yourself. Knowing where the different regions, parts and joints are located can help you begin to perceive and control your posture and movement better.

Here I am emphasizing the skeletal or bony aspects. Remember, though, that all the other kinds of tissues of the NMS system are also included. In addition, the major organ systems of the body are contained within this framework.

The Lower Back

We have gradually narrowed our focus from the organism-as-a-whole to the neuro-musculo-skeletal system, from the entire movement chain to the central axis of the body framework. We now have some context for looking at the structure and function of the lower back (lumbar area), while staying aware of these larger aspects.

The lower back is the most common trouble site for activity-related problems of the spine. A bit less than two-thirds of such problems are localized here, especially in the lowest segments. A bit more than a third of problems occur in the neck. Only a small percentage of problems occur in the upper back, the thoracic spine area.[5]

In Figure 5.5, you can see a simplified diagram of the lumbar vertebrae (back bones) and associated parts of the spine.

As I mentioned before, the lower back consists of five lumbar vertebrae and their related tissues. A good way to look at the spine is to see that it is made up of functional units known as *motion segments*. A motion segment consists of two adjacent vertebral bones and their related nerves, joints, ligaments, discs and muscles.

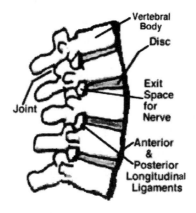

Figure 5.5 — Lumbar Vertebrae

Bones

The *vertebral body*, which makes up the main bony mass of a single lumbar vertebra, sits in front (*anteriorly*). This merges into a ring of bone called the *vertebral arch* (see Figure 5.6). The vertebral arch extends to the rear (*posteriorly*). Bony extensions also jut out along either side of the arch.

The vertebral body and arch together form a hole. When the vertebrae are 'stacked' on top of each other, the holes form a tube-like space called the *spinal canal*. The spinal canal contains the spinal cord.

Bony asymmetries—static deviations from a geometrically 'normal' alignment of the vertebrae—appear normal and do not necessarily mean that someone will have painful symptoms.

Nerves

The spinal cord provides the machinery for the lower levels of nervous system control related to basic motor output and sensation. It starts at the base of the brain and ends at about the level of the first lumbar bone (L1). When the spinal cord gets injured during serious trauma or in the case of serious medical problems, paralysis and loss of sensation can occur.

At each level from neck to lower back, spinal nerves come out of the cord, carrying motor and sensory fibers to the trunk and limbs. The spinal nerves also carry *autonomic fibers* that regulate glands and the smooth muscles of the organs, including the heart and blood vessels. Each nerve exits through a hole formed at each side of adjoining vertebrae. Since the spinal cord actually ends at the level of the L1 vertebra, spinal nerves below this level hang down within the spinal canal in a bundle called the *cauda equina* (Latin for horse's tail) before exiting along the sides between the vertebrae.

Joints

Two adjacent vertebrae have synovial joints located along each side (see Figure 5.1). In the lumbar spine, the bony surfaces of these joints allow mostly flexion (forward bending) and extension (backward bending). Practitioners of spinal manipulation may feel for increased or decreased movements in these joints. While this kind of testing can provide useful information at times, it cannot in itself determine the site or nature of a back problem.

Ligaments

Various ligaments not only reinforce the front and back outer portions of the disc but also connect the other bony parts of the motion segment (see Figure 5.5). These include the *anterior longitudinal ligament*, a broad fibrous band that runs along the anterior (front) part of the motion segment. The *posterior longitudinal ligament* supports the posterior (back) part of the vertebral body and disc. In the lumbar spine, it is not as broad as the anterior ligament. Especially along its sides (laterally) it does not cover either the vertebral body or the disc completely. This may explain why the posterior part of the disc is more vulnerable to mechanical stresses.

Discs

Intervertebral discs sit between each vertebral body starting in the upper to mid-neck and ending at the lower lumbar spine. Discs allow movement and serve as weight-bearing and shock-absorbing cushions for the spine.

The whole spine normally has twenty-one discs, which make up about a quarter of its length in adults.[6] The first disc is located between the second and third cervical vertebrae, the last between the fifth lumbar and first sacral vertebrae. Because each disc is located between adjacent vertebral bodies it can be classified as a separate joint composed of a special kind of cartilage. The disc is reinforced by ligaments in front and back and is separated from the vertebrae above and below it by cartilage *endplates*. Figure 5.6 shows a top-down view of a lumbar disc.

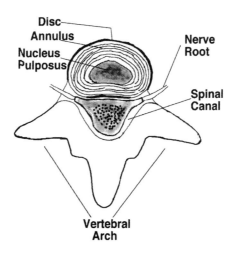

Figure 5.6 - Disc Structure

Internally, the disc is composed of a concentric outer layer of strong, stretchable connective tissue, called the *annulus*. Near its center the disc has a semi-fluid gel-like structure called the *nucleus pulposus* which contains large molecules that attract water. The enclosed fluid disc acts like a pressurized container that can accommodate movement and absorb shocks. After the first years of life, especially once we develop upright posture, the blood supply to the disc disappears. By the time we reach adulthood, the disc is the largest structure in our bodies that lacks a direct blood supply. Since it contains cells that require nutrients and give off waste products, the disc must exchange fluids with the surrounding tissues.

The weight of the body compresses the discs so that much of their fluid content moves into surrounding tissues. Depending on our age, we can lose as much as 18 millimeters of height in the course of a day. This equals about 1% of body height.[7] This loss of height can be accentuated or reduced by the amount of weight that we carry or whether we spend some time lying down.

When we are non-weight bearing, especially during the length of a night's sleep, fluids are reabsorbed. As a result, by the time we get up in the morning, we are usually taller than we were before we went to bed.

In the erect standing position, with the normal spinal curves, forces on the disc tend to be the most symmetrical, or evenly balanced. Different positions and movements, wherein the spinal curves either increase or decrease and reverse, tend to create asymmetrical pressures on the disc. Depending on the direction of this force, the shape of the disc and the position of the fluid nucleus inside of it will change as shown in Figure 5.7.[8]

During flexion (forward bending), the anterior part of the disc gets compressed, the posterior ligament gets tensed and the nucleus shifts to the back. During extension (backward bending), the opposite occurs with compression of the posterior part of the disc and shifting of the nucleus to the front. Bending towards the side tends to move the nucleus towards the opposite direction.

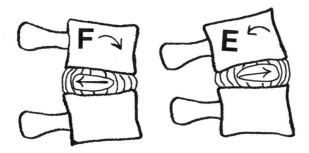

Figure 5.7 - Movements Within Disc

As we get older, we dry out. The water content of the disc tends to decrease. The nucleus becomes less distinct from its outer covering, which develops cracks and fissures. Since the disc material has no direct circulation, it does not regenerate. Cracks, fissures and other minor damage are repaired, not with new disc material, but with fibrous connective tissue. As a result of these changes, the disc space may shrink. This process, called "disc degeneration," continues into old age.

Since bone is a living changing tissue, changes to the surrounding bone also tend to occur. Nuclear material may push into the surrounding vertebral bodies. Movements within the disc that create persistent tensions on spinal ligaments may cause tensions on the attached bone as well. As a result, bony ridges called *osteophytes* may form that can be seen on x-rays.

Interestingly enough, spine researchers consider these changes part of the normal biological process of aging. Although they may be associated with reduced range of movement, they are not necessarily pathological or painful. If they were, we would expect the oldest among us to have the most back pain. This is not the case. Though elderly people may have posture and movement-related problems of their own, most acute lower back problems occur in those around 30 to 55 years of age. What could account for this?

During this prime time for back pain, the drying up and cracking of the disc continues to occur. However, movement within the disc is still possible. What may occur is that after being compressed, the discs of people in this age group tend to expand more rapidly and with greater pressure than those of either younger or older people. This may not be a problem unless our usual posture-movement pattern keeps us in a condition of asymmetrical pressure for too long, for example sitting for long periods of time.

After a continuous period of this kind, which combines compression with assymetrical positioning, the gel-like nuclear material will have shifted out of its neutral position. Pieces of this stuff may even get pushed into one or more cracks inside the disc. This substance may then expand and remain in the place where it has gotten pushed, similar to the way that a piece of material can get stuck or displaced inside of a hinge.

Movements which require the disc material to shift again may not allow this displaced material to change position quickly enough. Instead, the joint and surrounding tissues will experience abnormal stress, with pain and loss of movement resulting. This process has been called "intradiscal displacement." [9]

Muscles

When someone with lower back pain presents himself bent forwards in pain, unable to bring himself erect, a physician or other practitioner may feel the back muscles hardened in contraction. The patient may also find them tender to the touch. It is easy to conclude that the muscles are "in spasm" and are the source of pain. However, attributing pain to the back muscles may at times be mistaken.

First of all, when pain does get attributed to mucle spasm, the back muscles are often not in spasm. If they were, the person bent over in pain would not be bending forwards. In spasm, the back muscles would pull the person into an extended (backward bent) position, which is seldom seen in acute low back conditions.

In this kind of situation, what seems more likely to be happening is the following: If a displacement, say within the disc, obstructs joint movement, the person may feel forced to bend forwards as a way of holding or guarding the area in order to reduce pain. The back muscles will then automatically kick in to hold the person up, as they do with anyone bending forwards.[10]

Displacements can sometimes be resolved quickly, in a matter of minutes, by specific positions and movements or by joint manipulation. When this happens, not only can the person stand erect but also the muscles no longer feel hardened in contraction. Touching the muscles no longer hurts, either. There is no way that a muscle strain, which would involve at least some microscopic tearing of muscle fibers with subsequent bleeding, inflammation, etc., could resolve so quickly.

In this case, it seems unlikely that the back muscles themselves generate pain. However, the back muscles still have importance in the cause and prevention of lower back pain. This is because of the way they affect the movements of the spine and so affect other tissues.

There are many muscles that affect movements in the lumbar spine. I won't list them individually. In general, they include various anterior (front) abdominal muscles and posterior back muscles. The muscles in the back connect one or more motion segments of the spine. There are also muscles connecting the torso to both the upper and lower limbs. These also have an effect on the movement and posture of the spine.

Muscles tend to work in pairs that oppose one another. When one set of muscles is shortening, another set on the opposite side of the joint will lengthen. Muscles may work most efficiently when they first lengthen before they contract and shorten. In part this explains the windup of a baseball pitcher. If a muscle is chronically held in either too shortened or too lengthened a state, it will not function at its best. Muscles work best at their resting length, which can be slightly more stretched than ordinary. [11]

In general, we can classify muscles into physiological *flexors* and *extensors*. The flexors lie to the front of the spinal column from the neck down and the extensors lie along the back of the spinal column and along the backs of the thighs and legs. The extensors are sometime called *antigravity muscles* because they typically support the upright standing position against the pull of gravity.

In addition, these same muscles also seem to be laid out in diagonal patterns. In the torso, the muscles that affect the movements of the back form what anatomist Raymond Dart called a "double-spiral." Starting with the deep abdominal muscles along one side, a diagonal or spiral can be traced into the more superficial muscles on the opposite side. This in turn spirals around into a diagonal arrangement of the extensor muscles of the back. Diagonals can be traced on both sides, thus forming the "double spiral" described by Dart, that follows a path that he traced from the pelvis to the skull.

These spiral connections account for the abilities we have not only to flex and extend but also to rotate, bend sideways, etc. According to Dart, this non-typical way of looking at muscular arrangements may explain some of the curious postural distortions and fixations that can occur involving multiple areas of the body. [12]

Summary — Your Lengthening Spine

Your neuro-musculo-skeletal system functions as a whole even as you focus on one part. Your lower back takes part in a movement chain that includes the other segments of the spine as well as the limbs. As an important link in the movement chain, what happens in your lower back affects the rest of your spine and limbs. What happens in these other areas can, in turn, affect how your lower back functions.

Dynamic posture remains a matter of coordination of the system as a whole. This depends more on awareness than on the length and strength of your muscles. Therefore, awareness of the connections among the various parts of the movement chain will provide you with a more effective coordination of effort and a greater efficiency of movement than stretching and strengthening exercises for a particular area or part.

Your spine as a whole functions as part of your 'anti-gravity' system. The resistance of your spine to compression and other forces is assisted by the presence of its normal curves, the optimal length of postural muscles (especially the extensors) and the cushioning effects of the discs, among other factors. Spending more of your time functioning at full stature helps your antigravity system.

As noted, the disc does not have its own blood supply. As we age, its ability to move and its resistance to mechanical stresses tend to lessen. Reduced movement and postural monotony (which reduce circulation) can accelerate these changes. Maintaining asymmetrical positions can also distort the motion segments of the spine. To promote the optimal functioning of your spine, getting out of distorted asymmetrical positions as often as possible seems necessary. Postural variety, by balancing periods of activity and rest, compression and decompression, will help you to accomplish this.

The anatomy and physiology discussed in this chapter provide the beginnings of a basis for some standards for the proper use and functioning of your back; I can perhaps summarize this in one phrase: "a lengthening spine."

Ron Dennis writes:

The attainment of poise is ...a matter of learning the art of lengthening. Lengthening means pre-eminently that in

standing, sitting, walking, bending, or in any activity whatever, one must prevent both unnecessary muscular effort
and the very common distortions of the natural curves of
the spine.[13]

You'll benefit by keeping your lengthening spine in your
awareness, as we go on in the next chapter to examine injury
and pain in relation to the back.

Chapter 6

The Pain in Sprain...

Why does it hurt? That's probably a question many people ask themselves when they suffer from back, neck or other pain. In some ways it's not a very useful question to consider for very long since the 'why' often implies a kind of awfulizing and catastrophizing attitude that can get in the way of finding solutions and getting on with your life.

On another broader level, however, that question may bring us to consider why anyone has pain. What possible biological purpose could there be for experiencing pain?

The answer to why we feel pain seems obvious at first. The ability to experience pain warns us and protects us from damage. It leads us to reduce or eliminate our discomfort. But although pain can be useful in this way, the pain warning system works far from perfectly.

Some people with serious illnesses like cancer may not feel any pain as their problems develop. Although not inevitable, pain often occurs in such cases at the end stage of the illness when it would no longer seem to serve as a useful warning.[1]

Other people like soldiers in combat, accident survivors and disaster victims may not feel immediate pain despite serious injuries. In the heat of the moment of dealing with the battle or the accident, attention may not focus on personal damage as much as on escaping with one's life or helping fellow soldiers or accident victims.[2]

Experiments with hypnosis and placebos like sugar pills also indicate that the amount of pain does not necessarily correspond with the extent of injury. The use of these approaches indicates that physiological states and tissue reactions may sometimes relate, in part, to suggestion, expectation and psychological state.[3]

In other cases, some people are believed to have *psychogenic pain*. Such pain may be considered by some to have a psychological origin without tissue injury. The person is believed to be expressing internal conflicts and personal problems in the language of bodily distress.[4]

People may also experience pain long after an injury has healed, when damage is no longer impending or occurring. The phantom limb pains often experienced by people who have lost a limb are a good example of this type of process. Some chronic back and neck problems may also involve this kind of condition. This may have something to do with damage to nerves which can then become hyperexcitable, or to other nervous system mechanisms.

The phantom limb phenomenon also brings out the point that we often inaccurately locate the source of pain. You need not have had an amputation to experience *referred pain*, where pain is projected to—experienced in—an area of the body other than the site of injury.[5]

As we grow up we learn to associate the site of an injury with a specific area of the skin that we can see or touch. We do this because we do not have visual and tactile experience with areas deep within our bodies or even deep in our muscles and joints. We may thus project or interpret input from such areas as coming from another part of the body (the skin) that shares a common nerve pathway, but with which we are more familiar.[6]

For example, pains felt in the muscles of the buttocks or down the thigh may have their actual source deep in the joints of the lower back. This can be confusing but, fortunately, referred pain patterns have been mapped out. This can help health professionals pinpoint the pain source.

In various ways, then, the pain warning system appears less than perfect. Nonetheless, there does remain some cause-effect relation between pain and injury. Pain can warn us that damage is impending or occurring. The changes that we observe in relation to the pain we feel can give us some indicators about what to do and what not to do. We can learn how to heed the messages of pain more carefully.

What 'Is' Pain?

Pain is not something in a bone, muscle, joint, etc. "The pain in sprain is mainly in the brain!"[7] In other words, your nervous system constructs the complex psycho-physical experience of pain. The International Association for the Study of Pain defines it as *"an unpleasant sensory and emotional experience associated with actual or potential tissue damage, or described in terms of such damage."*[8]

A useful framework for understanding some of the more specific mechanisms of pain perception is the Gate Theory of Melzack and Wall, first formulated in the 1960s.[9]

According to the Gate Theory, messages from receptors sensitive to noxious input travel along certain nerve fibers into various transmitting cells in the spinal cord. These transmitting cells then send their own signals to higher levels of the nervous system/brain and to other cells that signal muscles to contract.

Transmitting cells are influenced not only by 'pain' input but also by the input of other sensory receptors from skin, muscles and joints. These other receptors are called mechanical receptors and convey signals related to touch, movement and other non-noxious stimulation.

Transmitting cells also get input from cells located in another part of the spinal cord that serve as the 'gates' of the theory. These gates can shut down or open up the transmission of potential pain messages.

Both the 'pain' and touch/movement messages branch into these gates, as well as to the transmitting cells. 'Pain' messages inhibit ('close') the gates and touch/movement messages facilitate ('open') the gates.

If a gate gets opened sufficiently by touch/movement signals, it will inhibit a transmitting cell from sending potential pain messages to higher levels, in spite of input indicating damage. In this way, a sufficient amount of peripheral touch and movement stimulation can reduce or prevent the experience of pain. This explains in part the effects of massage and movement (manipulation or exercise) as well as heat and cold in reducing pain.

The entire system of gating and transmission cells also receives inhibitory and facilitating input from the cerebral cortex and inhibitory input from the brainstem. The existence of these higher-level inputs provides a way to begin to explain how beliefs, attitudes, anxiety, hypnosis, etc., can influence the experience of pain.

The Chemistry of Pain

The nervous system reactions discussed above are mediated by a complex chemistry. This bio-chemical aspect relates not only to how we deal with pain but also to how we think, feel and act in general.

Chemical messengers called neuropeptides are necessary for the transmission of signals from one nerve cell to another. These neuropeptides are related to hormones. They affect and are affected by other organ systems of the body, including the immune system. The neuropeptides and the hormones can be considered the communication molecules of the organism.

Around 1970, scientists gradually became aware of the possible existence of receptors on nerves and other organs for these kinds of chemicals. Receptors for morphine, a powerful plant-derived pain killer, were discovered in various sites in the brain and in other organs.

Scientist reasoned that, if such receptors existed, they did not evolve in order to fit the morphine molecule. There must be some naturally occurring substance in our brains similar in structure to morphine. Eventually, several such substances, which work not only for the pain control but also for the cardiovascular and other systems, were discovered and given the name *endorphins* for endogenous (inner) morphine.

Endorphin receptors exist in the 'gate' areas of the spinal cord. In the brain, endorphin receptors are wide-spread, although they are particularly concentrated in the limbic system (especially involved with emotions) and in an area in the midbrain. This last area sends powerful inhibitory signals to the spinal cord. It has many connections with other areas of the brain and may account for some of the effects of placebos and hypnosis since electrical stimulation of this area results in wide-spread pain reduction.[10]

This undoubtedly is part of a larger complex system that affects pain perception. It can be affected, in turn, by disease and injury, drugs, sensory-motor stimulation, anxiety, expectations, learning and personality, among other factors.

The neurological circuits and neurochemical connections discussed here are related to what you do and how you think and feel. They likely evolved because they enhanced our ancestors' ability to survive—to mobilize themselves to fight or flee from danger and further damage. Each one of us has inherited what Melzack and Wall call these "natural resources in the brain."[11]

The Experience of Pain

You don't need to understand these neurological and neurochemical connections in great detail. It is sufficient to know that they exist and that your experience of pain is intimately related to them. Let us look more closely at your nervous system experience of pain (what you do and feel) illustrated in Figure 6.1.

Let's start at Level I. Something happens in your lower back. Let's say that you bend forwards unexpectedly and a bone, disc, joint, ligament, muscle or nerve suddenly gets stretched, compressed or even injured to some degree (there may or may not be injury).

At Level II, the immediate sensory impact, nerve fibers in your back can be stimulated in response to the sudden mechanical pressure or pull. If injury has occurred, chemicals resulting from inflammation may stimulate nerve receptors. However, at this point, you do not yet have an experience of pain. The arrow from II to III stands for the nervous system processes in the spinal cord and brain involving the gate cells, transmitting cells, etc.

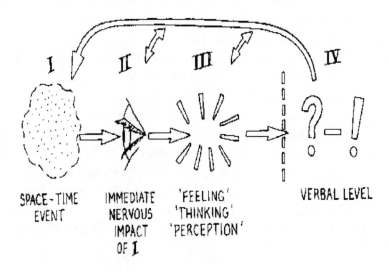

SPACE-TIME EVENT   IMMEDIATE NERVOUS IMPACT OF **I**   'FEELING' 'THINKING' 'PERCEPTION'   VERBAL LEVEL

Figure 6.1 — Nervous System Processing of Pain[12]

Level III represents the even more complex nervous system processes of your non-verbal experience (what you later call "pain"). If you feel some discomfort in your back or in some other part of your body right now, just notice it. If not, for the purpose of experiment (you are a personal scientist after all!), pinch your finger. What do you feel? Whatever words you then say about it, such as "ouch!" or "it's painful!" etc., *are not* the experience itself.

Distinguishing your non-verbal pain experience from the way that you talk about it, and learning to observe your pain and other symptoms better, can help you deal more effectively with your symptoms.

With Level IV, we arrive at the verbal level. At this level you describe your experience in words, i.e., "flickering, sharp, dull," etc. Your words may involve judgements and conclusions about your experience, i.e., "dreadful, unbearable, vicious," etc., or "Hmm, perhaps that's a warning, better change how I'm sitting."

What you describe and talk about at Level IV partly depends upon the stress or injury at Level I and your Levels II and III processing of it. How you talk about the pain also reflects how you evaluate your previous experience. For example, you might say things like "How stupid to injure my back again" or "Another onset, too bad! What's the best way to deal with it now?" Which general attitude may be more constructive in the long run?

According to general semanticists, Level IV is not something 'mental' apart from the physical. Rather, your interpretation or evaluation involving language qualifies as a nervous system event as much as what happens on Levels II and III.

Your Level IV interpretation is also not the linear end point of some pain-causing stimulus. Rather, the entire experience of pain, like most other human experiences, is very much part of an ongoing process of circular causation.

This circular or cyclic process of causation is shown in the looping arrows on top of the diagram that go from the 'higher' to 'lower' levels of reacting. In practical terms, this means that your evaluation of your back pain (the meaning you give to it), which includes how you talk about it to yourself, can shape your ongoing behavior and your experience of pain. This means, among other things, that anticipating pain may make you more sensitive to it.

I do *not* say here that your back pain is just a matter of what you believe and how you behave. I do say that your experience of pain does not simply depend upon some immediate 'noxious' input. Your experience of pain, as indicated in Figure 6.1, depends upon many levels of nervous system functioning. These levels can involve beliefs, attitudes, moods, attention, etc., as well as various drugs and other chemicals, and different types of sensory stimulation and movement, among other factors.

Many Paths to Feeling Better

In this chapter I have touched on the fact that pain is not simply a function of injury. Many factors enter into whether and to what extent you will experience pain. Many influences bear on whether the 'gates' of the spinal cord will open or close to let nerve signals become painful experiences. Therefore, it is likely that many different kinds of treatment, working on different levels in different ways, can help you to feel less pain.

It is useful to know that there are many ways of dealing with your pain. The advantage of using activity-related (posture-movement) approaches to deal with activity-related pain is that you deal directly with a significant source of your back pain problem.

As I discuss in greater detail later, non-damaging movement can often usefully reduce the chemical irritants that accumulate after a musculoskeletal injury to the back (or neck, etc.).

Properly guided movements (exercises) may also help resolve activity-related pain caused by shortened muscles and stiff joints, as well as pain resulting from the kind of intervertebral joint displacements discussed in the previous chapter.

Non-damaging movement also provides peripheral stimulation that can help open the spinal cord gates that turn off the further transmission of potential pain signals.

Improved posture-movement habits provide a non-irritating environment for the muscles and joints to heal without further damage.

In addition, doing something to take control of your painful symptoms in itself has positive benefits. Taking action for your own well-being provides a sense of efficacy and self-confidence. For one thing, it gets your attention away from simply dwelling upon your symptoms. As neurologist Barry Wyke has pointed out, you should not overlook the power of "ensuring cerebral disregard" (distraction).[13]

In the next chapter, we take a deeper look at the psychology of control and its relation to pain and posture.

Chapter 7

You Control Your Pain and Posture

You are not a victim of circumstance, at the mercy of your painful symptoms. Rather, you can control your back pain. As already shown, you often can control your pain by changing your posture and movement.

Such control is not perfect. Nonetheless, you have probably not come close to exhausting the possibilities for gaining control of your symptoms. In this chapter, I explain what some behavioral scientists have learned about the process of controlling your experience.

Consistent Results, Variable Actions

Although they are not immune to the laws of physics, living creatures, including you, are not like inanimate objects that simply respond to a push or a kick by moving a predictable amount. Unlike a rock, you move under your own power.

Neither are you a stimulus-response machine, destined to react in a set, reflexive way. Rather, you have purposes, choices, options. When pushed you may resist, push back or decide to yield.

In order to survive as a dynamic system functioning as an organism-as-a-whole-in-an-environment, you transact with a changing and turbulent world. You take action and evaluate the results in order to maintain a certain set of relatively constant conditions inside and outside yourself. You attempt to get what you want to satisfy your needs.

Imagine a world that always gives you what you want and need. Would you have to act or to perceive the results of your actions? Probably not!

However, as you know, we do not live in such a world. Instead, the changing, turbulent world in which we live is full of disturbances. It not only doesn't give you what you want but often gives you what you don't want — things like back pain! Life, it has been said, is what happens while you were making other plans.

To get what you want, despite whatever disturbances occur, you need to know what result you desire. You also need to perceive current reality, what presently is going on inside and outside your skin.[1] Psychologist William T. Powers writes:

> The general rule is that if you want to control something [achieve a particular result you desire], you have to perceive it. This doesn't mean just perceiving that something exists,...It means perceiving exactly the aspect of the world that is supposed to be under control.[2]

In this way you can adjust your actions to give you the particular experiences you want.

This ability to adjust your actions has importance. You pursue particular consistent perceivable results through variable actions. Powers considers this a central defining feature of behavior. For example, picture that you're driving and managing to keep your car inside your intended lane.[3] You are probably not conscious of what particular muscle contractions you make. Instead you are controlling for a particular perceivable result, staying inside the lane. There may be cross winds, bumps on the road, pressure changes in your tires, among other things. To achieve your desired perceivable result, you must counter these moment to moment disturbances with your varying actions.

You sometimes may move the wheel or sometimes hold it steady in one position. In either case, your moment to moment motor output, which cannot be programmed in advance, serves the ongoing purpose of continuing to give you the consistent experience of staying between the lines of the lane (if that's what you want to experience). Though your visible actions may appear similar from one time to the next, the exact particular actions you make at any one time must vary to take varying environmental conditions into account.

There are some regularities in the world and over time we tend to develop more or less stable systems of behavior, or habits, for getting what we want. So our visible actions, although variable, do have a certain consistency as well (hands on steering wheel, etc.). These habit systems develop pretty much unconsciously from trial and error.

Feedback Control

What I have been describing above is the operation of a negative feedback control system. In everything you do, you seek to control for the perceivable results you want to experience (for example, you may be reading this book in order to learn how to control your back pain and your related posture-movement habits).

The notion of feedback has been applied throughout physiology to understand how our body systems function to maintain a more-or-less steady internal state (the concept of homeostasis). Surprisingly, though, only a small group of scientists have comprehensively applied this notion to our external behavior. Many of them work in the field of *Perceptual Control Theory* (*PCT*) formulated by Powers and his associates.[4] As Richard J. Robertson, Ph.D., notes:

> Control theory is the most recent in a succession of names for the developing body of theory based on a feedback system paradigm. Other names are "cybernetic-psychology," "general feedback theory of human behavior," or simply, "systems theory psychology."[5]

Despite the complexities involved, the bare basics of a simple one-level negative feedback control system can be seen in Figure 7.1. This schematic model, along with the description which follows, explains the organization of a simple control system such as one that you are probably familiar with—a thermostat.[6]

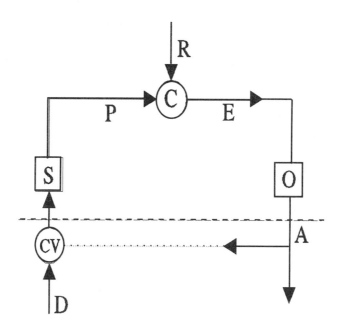

Figure 7.1 — A Negative Feedback Control System

Key to Negative Feedback Loop

1. The action or output **(A)** of the furnace **(0)** [output device],

2. The environment in which it acts, including disturbances **(D)** [The downward pointing arrow from O represents **A's** unintended consquences on the environment],

3. The temperature, the controlled variable **(CV)** influenced by both **A** and **D**, sensed or measured by the sensor **(S)** [The effect of **A** on **CV** constitutes the actual feedback.],

4. The perceptual signal **(P)** created by the sensor,

5. The internal standard or reference level of the 'desired' temperature **(R)**,

6. The comparison **(C)** and difference/error **(E)** between perception and reference which signals the furnace to produce an output, and so back to **1**, etc.

The activity of the thermostat-furnace system gets the controlled variable of temperature to the desired reference level. The system involves a circular or cyclic loop of causation from system to environment to system involving *feedback*, since the results of the system's actions affect the ongoing activity of the system. It is a *negative feedback* loop because the actions of the system exactly negate or counter whatever disturbances occur to move the controlled variable away from the 'desired' temperature.

The parts of this loop of causation happen all at once so that the ongoing output affects the sensed input at the same time that the sensed input affects the ongoing output. The internal standards of the thermostat have primary importance in determining what happens in the system.

A thermostat system is designed to control a variable in its environment, the temperature of the room. I label the temperature **CV** for *controlled variable*. The thermostat has a *sensor* (**S**) or input device that changes in a predictable and precise way in relation to the temperature. This sensor creates an ongoing *perceptual signal* inside the thermostat labeled **P**.

In an area inside the thermostat, labeled **C** for *comparator*, this perceptual signal gets compared with a reference, an internal standard, that has been set for the temperature. This *reference level*, labeled **R**, represents a goal state, an intended level for perceivable temperature. In the case of the thermostat, you create this reference level when you put the setting of your thermostat at 72 degrees (or whatever temperature pleases you) in order to create a toasty winter environment.

The difference between **R** and **P**, labeled **E**, is called the *error* of the system (a technical term for a normal part of a feedback systems operation). When the temperature is at 72 degrees or above, **E** = 0. In this case, there is no **E** signal and the furnace remains off. However, when the temperature measured by **S** goes below 72 degrees, **E** becomes a positive value and provides a signal to an *output* device (**O**), the furnace.

The furnace, in turn, acts on the environment of the house, including the room where the thermostat is located. Let's say it blows warm air through air ducts which feed into the rooms of the house. I label the action, which includes whatever operations occur inside the furnace, **A**. The activities of the furnace may, of course have other effects on the environment besides the intended one on the controlled variable.

In addition to the action of the furnace, there are many different external factors that affect the **CV**, the temperature of the room. The outside weather, drafts created when doors and windows open and close, people walking by, the number of people in the room, some other heat source near the thermostat, etc., all serve as *disturbances,* labeled **D**. These disturbances move **CV** away from the desired reference value **R**. The actions of the furnace must counter these influences.

Depending upon the reliability of the sensor and the sensitivity with which the system responds to error, the control system of thermostat and furnace may keep the room temperature at a steady 72 degrees despite any disturbances that occur.

Behavior: The Control of Perception

According to Control Theory, the thermostat–furnace–temperature control system has been designed by engineers to do what you and other living things do all the time (though often imperfectly): *control your perceptions*. As Robertson notes:

> ...a profound consequence of this theory for psychology is the implication that living organisms do not control their environments by controlling their outputs. They control their inputs—their 'perceptions'—as Powers states in the title of his book, *Behavior: The Control of Perception.*[7]

The system shown in Figure 7.1 controls its input. In other words, it keeps the perception (**P**) of temperature matching the reference (**R**) for desired temperature. **P** is kept equal to **R** even when there are disturbances (**D**) like drafts and people that would tend to push **P** away from **R** (the desired value for **P**).

You function as a perceptual control system. Like the thermostat I've described, you act to control what you perceive— your perceptual input. However, humans (unlike thermostats) set their own **R** values. This is autonomy. People decide what they want to perceive (they set the **R** in their brains) and act to make their perceptions continuously match **R**.

When you change **R** (change what you want), the perception **P** changes right along with the wanted **R**. So control of perception means that you are continuously deciding what you want to perceive and are acting to perceive it. If you are not perceiving what you want to perceive, then there is a failure of control.

You obviously are a lot more complicated than a simple thermostat. According to the PCT model, your nervous system is made up of a huge number of control systems arranged in a hierarchy of at least 11 levels of nerve networks that intercommunicate.[8] Each level involves different and increasingly complex kinds of perception. The names of these 11 perceptual levels, moving from the most basic to the most complex, are *intensity, sensation, configuration, transition, event, relationship, category, sequence, program, principle* and *system*. To get a sense of what intercommunication among these levels might look like, imagine a network of tiny Christmas lights linked together and glittering off and on in intricate patterns.

The PCT model proposes that each successive level of perception gets constructed from the previous lower levels. We control our perceptions at each of these levels in the way that the thermostat controls the temperature of the room.

At the lowest level of control, the output of the system directly results in muscle contractions that, when combined with environmental disturbances, result in your visible movements and activities.

Your actions are significantly determined by the higher level perceptions/references (beliefs, principles, values, etc.) that operate in you. The direct output of any of these higher levels of control is not to the muscles directly. Rather, higher levels provide the reference signals to lower levels of control. As a consequence, your yearning for chocolate ice cream may eventually result in any number of different actions, such as driving, bicycling or walking to an ice cream shop.

Reorganization and Learning

So far I've described the organization of a hierarchical control system already present and operating. Except for some basic 'reflexes', you are not born with control loops at any of these levels. How do they develop? How do you learn to control the important variables of your life?

PCT theorists propose the existence of an innate, genetically determined system called the *Intrinsic Reorganizing System*. The Intrinsic Reorganizing System underlies the operation of all of the 11 levels noted above and also works on negative feedback principles.

The Intrinsic Reorganizing System includes the system of basic needs that you have at birth. These needs involve preset reference levels for such physiological and biochemical quantities as blood sugar, oxygen, carbon dioxide, etc.

Various sensors in your nervous system/brain, especially in the hypothalamus, monitor these levels, thus providing feedback to your Reorganizing System. This system may also monitor internal conflicts among the various levels of the behavioral control hierarchy as well as continued errors beyond a certain amount at any particular level.

According to the Reorganization model, feedback regarding your intrinsically controlled states such as blood sugar or oxygen gets compared to the reference levels for those states. Any difference between the two generates an intrinsic error signal that directs a message to your 11-level behavioral control hierarchy to reorganize.

Reorganization basically functions by trial and error. As Robertson points out:

> An 'organizing-reorganizing' system activated by rising error signals within the intrinsic system, functions similarly to the random signal generator used by cybernetic engineers to inject miscellaneous neural impulses into the control hierarchy, thereby arbitrarily resetting reference signals and disrupting homeostasis.[9]

Neural connections get altered. Reference levels, perceptual signals, relations within the hierarchy, etc., all have the potential to get changed. The rate of reorganization depends on the amount of intrinsic error present. The visible results of all of this will be seen in changes in what you do. Presumably, reorganization will continue until the error of your intrinsic system equals zero. New perceptual control circuits (habits) will get created in such a trial and error process by their ability to reduce intrinsic error. Powers writes:

> Reorganization theory relies on a model of the internal workings of the organism. It says that we learn in order to satisfy internal needs, and that we stop varying the way we behave in a given environment (although we don't stop behaving) when those needs are met.[10]

Some interesting implications follow from seeing learning as a reorganization process. For one thing, this viewpoint implies that problems and obstacles constitute opportunities for learning. Difficult people, frustrations, mistakes and problems, including the pains that you feel, may serve as 'teachers'. In his book *Wholistic Healing*, Dr. Elan Z. Neev writes:

> One of the best ways to Wholistic health is total acceptance of life as a series of lessons. This attitude will automatically remove much of the strain and stress of everyday life and of the painful experiences of the past or the dread of tomorrow....every experience is an opportunity for learning and growth, every problem, mistake, failure, pain, and obstacle is beneficial if we are willing to learn from it....Look for the blessings in disguise, even if the disguise is excellent![11]

Seeing learning as reorganization also means that no one can teach anything to someone else in the sense of simply 'pouring content' into a waiting, empty 'container'. What you learn will result from your own reorganization process—what you put together in your own somewhat unique way. This cannot be entirely programmed by someone else. At best a teacher or a book can only facilitate learning for you by creating the conditions for your reorganization process.

Attention may have an important role in this process. Attention seems to function as a way of focusing reorganization on the particular areas of experience that will most likely have the greatest effect on reducing the intrinsic error present. In this way, the reorganization process does not have to be totally random. Your skill in directing your attention and calmly observing what is going on (functioning as a personal scientist) can help you direct your learning process more effectively.

Emotions or feelings can also be understood in relation to the intrinsic system. Emotions seem to correspond to our internal perceptions of our intrinsic state. When you are going through some sort of reorganization process, whether minor or major, you may feel varying levels of confusion, distress, anxiety, conflict, etc. It's important to understand that these kinds of feeling are normal. Accepting your feelings will allow your Reorganization System to work more efficiently as your "mind's repair kit," as social worker/educator Edward E. Ford calls it.[12] When you realize this, you can avoid additional distress created by feeling anxious about your anxiety and confused about your confusion when you are learning something new.

Controlling Pain

The experience of pain involves a continuous feedback control loop. The loop includes perception, desire and action at multiple levels of the nervous system. This has been implicitly recognized by others besides Perceptual Control psychologists. For example, pain scientist Patrick Wall writes:

Our understanding brains steadily combine all the available information from the outside world and within our own bodies with our personal and genetic histories. The outcomes are decisions or tactics and strategies that could be appropriate to respond to the situation. We use the word *pain* as shorthand for one of these groupings of relevant response tactics and strategies. Pain is not just a sensation but, like hunger and thirst, is an awareness of an action plan to be rid of it.[13]

Initially, your back pain may have started as an unintended consequence of controlling for some other variable, such as lifting a package, sitting too long on a plane, etc. At some point, your sensation of back pain became a variable you sought to control in its own right. If you have an ongoing back pain problem, it may now qualify as a poorly controlled variable.

Pain involves not just one thing but rather many dimensions of perception that vary (see Index Your Symptoms in Chapter 10). It can feel strong or weak, sharp or thick, short or long, etc. You can locate it in different parts of your body, e.g., your lower or upper back, on either side, down your leg, etc. When you control a perception, you pick the perception that you want and try to act in a way that produces that perception. So if you want less pain anywhere, you have to act to bring the different dimensions of the perception to their desired state.

As indicated in the previous chapter, there are many pathways that may be used to deal with pain. Your efforts to reduce your pain may have made use of some of them. However, you may not have taken full advantage of posture-movement methods of pain control.

This book suggests kinds of actions that you can take to influence your pain perceptions. If you have activity-related pain, you can reduce, change the location of and eliminate your symptoms by means of positions and movements. You can begin to change your posture-movement habits to reduce the stress on your back. Using these approaches, you can learn to judge whether what you are doing is changing your perception of pain in the way that you want.

Controlling Posture

Perceptual Control Theory (PCT) also relates to how you use yourself, your posture-movement habits, which can affect your back pain symptoms. PCT provides some possible explanations for how your habits developed. It also suggests guidelines for learning to improve these habits.

A major portion of your "self-sensing" (proprioceptive) perception system monitors your body position and movements. This system includes numerous sensory receptors in the muscles, tendons and joints, as well as the inner ear.

As you developed from babyhood, one of the first areas that you learned to perceive and control was your own body. Your body use developed more or less by trial and error learning through a process of reorganization. This process of reorganization did not necessarily lead to the optimal way of using yourself. Rather this trial and error process resulted in your tending to act like a short-term opportunist. It led to whatever behavior worked for the moment, e.g., catching the ball tossed to you, keeping from falling down, or picking up a heavy box.

In this way you formed a more or less stable system of unconscious posture-movement habits controlled by negative feedback—a postural set point (homeostasis).[14] This set point, which became your standard of body use, may explain the resistence that you experience when beginning to change bad postural habits which have come to feel 'right'. Your short-term opportunism continued as you got older and focused ever less attention on the lower levels of the hierarchy of behavior, especially those perceptions involving body use. As a result, your body use got put on the 'back burner' of your awareness.

This is very much what happened to F.M. Alexander, who I wrote about in Chapter 4. Alexander sought to achieve a short-term perceivable result (his end), projecting his voice to the farthest corner of the performance hall. He perceived success in doing that. However, he did not at first notice the fact that the tense and awkward way in which he did it (his means) led to strain and hoarseness in the long run.

If you successfully pick up the package you want to lift by means of bending awkwardly, you may not notice that the tense and uncoordinated way you do it may lead to strain and pain in the long run.

In other words, for any particular perceivable result you seek to bring about (your end or goal), you, like most if not all other humans, naturally tend to ignore the means (process) that you use to achieve them. For example, if you carry a bag with a shoulder strap are you aware of whether or not you unecessarily raise your shoulder to do it? You (like most, if not all, other humans) tend to tune out unintended consequences—unless, for example, bodily pain and strain feels severe and lasting enough to signal intrinsic error and 'demand' reorganization.

Initially, F. M. Alexander was not aware of how his use was creating his vocal problems. People with back and neck pain and repetitive strain are often not initially aware of how their body use affects these problems. Recognizing that your problems may be affected by how you are using yourself is an important first step towards doing something constructive about it.

Perceiving this relation can narrow the amount of trial and error required to develop more effective control of your posture and pain. For example, a student of mine, a massage therapist, always had a pain in his back while doing dishes. The pain vanished when he learned to fold his body rather than bend it (see Chapter 13). He quickly was able to apply this to other activities that had previously brought discomfort, e.g. bending over his massage table.

The bottom line here is this: You have many ways to move and you can relearn new ones. Although you tend not to focus on them, your own actions (though not usually the individual muscle contractions) are perceivable aspects of your environment that you can direct your attention to and control. Once you see the particular relations among posture, movement and pain that hold for you, it's possible to begin to view your bodily use as an area of interest to explore and change.

Part III

Therapy Solutions

...we need comfort, support, recognition and help
if we are to make the best of our days in pain.
– Patrick Wall[1]

Chapter 8

Diagnosing Back Pain

Most episodes of back pain represent activity-related (mechanical) problems that can improve with time, appropriate pain control and posture-movement approaches. Such problems include what Waddell calls "simple backache," as well as many cases of "nerve root pain," wherein leg pain is associated with evidence of injury to a single nerve root. Leg pain, sometimes called "sciatica," may also get referred from a severe backache without nerve root involvement.[1]

If this is the first time that you have had a significant back problem or if your symptoms are different from previous episodes and you have not received a diagnosis, I suggest that you go to a medical doctor (an internist or family practitioner will often do). As I mentioned in Chapter 2, specific diagnosis of back pain is controversial. However, a general screening diagnosis which reasonably separates activity-related problems from other less likely but more serious medical/surgical conditions can be readily done.[2] A physician who can perform such a screening can provide reasonable assurance that you do not have a serious medical or surgical disease. With that knowledge you can proceed more confidently and safely in pursuit of posture-movement solutions.

In order to diagnose your problem, your doctor will likely get a history—your story of the problem, how it started, what your pain is like, etc. He or she may also examine your back by inspecting it visually, observing your posture and manner of walking, as well as doing a more detailed spinal examination. Among other things, he or she may ask you to bend forwards, backwards and sideways, with one or two movements each, to assess the amount of movement you have and whether or not you have pain. He or she may test the muscles of your legs as well as your sensation and reflexes to see if there is any indication of a nerve root getting pinched. In some cases he or she may decide to do x-rays or other tests as well.

Red Flags

Only a small percentage of back problems result from serious disorders such as fractures, tumors, infections or inflammatory diseases.[3] These uncommon sources of back pain need to be detected before they can be treated effectively. Therefore, you should see a medical doctor if you can answer "yes" to one or more of the following questions. These are considered "red flags" that may indicate possible serious conditions that need to be looked into further.[4]

 • *Are you under the age of 20? Are you over the age of 55 and experiencing a first onset of back symptoms or different ones than usual?*

 • *Do you feel constant pain at rest or moving that does not improve with any positions or movements?*

 • *Do you have pain at night not relieved by medication?*

 • *Have your symptoms continued to worsen since they began?*

 • *Do you experience persistent restriction of spinal movements?*

 • *Do you have a major spinal deformity (are unable to straighten up or are twisted to one side) or notice any significant change in the appearance of your back?*

 • *Have you been in an accident, had a fall or experienced some other form of trauma?*

 • *Do you have pain, pins and needles or numbness in your leg or foot?*

 • *Do you notice weakness in your leg or foot?*

• *Have you suddenly lost bowel or bladder control or do you feel tingling or numbness around your groin and anus?* (If so, this requires immediate emergency medical attention!)

• *Do you feel generally unwell, experience a fever, or have unexplained weight loss?*

• *Do you have a past medical history of cancer, systemic steroid use, drug abuse or HIV?*

Below, I briefly discuss possible meanings of each of these "red flags."

Are you under the age of 20 ? Are you over the age of 55 and experiencing a first onset of back symptoms or different ones than usual? For those under the age of 20 or over 55, especially those who have never had a significant back problem before, x-rays and other tests may be needed to rule out more serious structural problems or diseases.

Do you feel constant pain at rest or moving that does not improve with any positions or movements? Do you have pain at night not relieved by medication? If you feel constant pain that does not seem to improve with changes in positioning or movement or that disturbs your sleep, these indicate the need for further investigation by your doctor. Your problems may involve a significant non-mechanical condition such as an inflammatory disease.

Have your symptoms continued to worsen since they began? Persistent or worsening pain should also get you to the doctor since this does not follow the expected pattern for the natural history of back pain.

Do you experience persistent major restriction of spinal movements? Do you have a severe spinal deformity (are unable to straighten up or are twisted to one side) or notice any significant change in the appearance of your back? Severe restrictions or deformities may indicate a problem beyond a simple backache. It may involve a major mechanical problem (like an extensive disc herniation) or some other medical or surgical condition that requires further investigation and help.

Have you been in an accident, had a fall or experienced some other form of trauma? Pain and difficulty moving after an accident or other trauma may mean no more than a sprain or strain. Although x-rays are no longer recommended for every complaint of spinal pain, they have a use when the doctor wants to rule out fractures and other more serious forms of injury. Depending on the type, extent and severity of your symptoms, your doctor may decide to do x-rays or some other form of diagnostic imaging.

Do you have pain, pins and needles or numbness in your leg or foot? Do you notice weakness in your leg or foot? Pain, pins and needles, numbness and weakness in the lower extremities may indicate that a nerve root has gotten compressed, most likely by a disc herniation. Impending or increasing neurological damage may also indicate a need for further study.

Have you suddenly lost bowel or bladder control or do you feel tingling or numbness around your groin and anus? A loss of bowel or bladder control can indicate a large disc herniation pressing against the bundle of nerves (the cauda equina) that provide sensation and motor control to these vital functions. A relatively rare occurrence, this indicates the need for immediate surgery, which can prevent permanent loss of control of these functions.

Do you feel generally unwell, experience a fever, or have unexplained weight loss? If you feel unwell or have a fever, your doctor may want to do further tests to rule out the rare possibilities of infection or an inflammatory illness.

Do you have a past medical history of cancer, systemic steroid use, drug abuse or HIV? A medical history of cancer, systemic steroid use, drug abuse or HIV does not mean that your back pain is necessarily caused by these. However, your doctor should know about such things, as they can be related to serious, though rare, spinal diseases.

I will repeat: even if none of these situations is present, I recommend that you see your medical doctor if you are experiencing your first significant episode of back pain and/or have not previously had your present symptoms diagnosed. If the probability of having more serious and relatively rare conditions has been reasonably ruled out, the doctor is likely to give you a general diagnosis of mechanical (activity-related) lower back pain. He or she will likely be able to prescribe medications that can help you to get through the episode with greater comfort. He or she may also provide you with some general postural advice and advice on activities and exercise. As I already noted in Chapter 2, such general advice may not always help you sufficiently to deal with your particular activity-related, posture-movement problem.

Activity-Related Pain and the Diagnostic Impasse

Simple activity-related back pain remains, as I have noted, one of the most common complaints that brings people to the doctor's office. Yet the attempt to get more specific about this general diagnosis has gotten stuck at an impasse which I already described in Chapter 2. I will further discuss the nature of that impasse here.

The word "diagnosis" comes from the Greek words "gnosis" for "seeing or knowing" and "dia" for "through." Thus "diagnosis" implies a kind of "seeing through" a particular set of observations or facts in order to infer an underlying, though not directly visible, cause or causes for a particular problem in a particular individual.

A physician or other health professional does tests and makes observations that allow her to make inferences about an underlying cause that she cannot directly observe. Biologist and medical educator M. L. J. Abercrombie describes diagnosis as "a process of *judgement*; that is, making a decision or conclusion on the basis of indications and probabilities" when the information is incomplete (no one ever has all of the information about anything).[5]

For example, a man falls while skiing. His foot spasms and twists and he can't put weight on it. He may or may not feel much pain. The emergency room doctor examines him with her unaided senses. She suspects a fracture based on her observations and her experience and knowledge of similar cases. Her tentative diagnostic inference of a fracture allows her to make predictions that can be tested, e.g., x-rays will show a fracture. This and other tests can then be done that support or bring into question what the doctor infers. A firmer diagnosis can be made which succeeds if it leads to effective treatment.

A basic set of assumptions for diagnosing musculoskeletal problems (a working theory) was formulated by James Cyriax, M.D.:

1. All pain arises from a lesion. [Some pain does not arise from a lesion, as I will show in Chapter 9.]

2. All treatment must reach the lesion.

3. All treatment must exert a beneficial effect on the lesion.[6]

A musculoskeletal lesion is defined as a pathological condition in a particular tissue, a muscle, joint, disc, ligament,etc. A fourth principle seems implicit here: the practitioner's goal should be to discover the tissue at fault so that a beneficial treatment can be given. This becomes the point of diagnosis.

Laslett points out two elements desirable in making a musculoskeletal diagnosis: First, where is it? This means identifying the specific anatomical site or tissue involved, i.e., muscle, joint, disc, etc. Second, what is it? This involves identifying the nature of the condition affecting the tissue, i.e., fracture, inflammation, activity-related problem, etc.[7]

Fractures and severe sprains, strains, dislocations, etc., are examples of musculoskeletal problems that can be specifically diagnosed very successfully as to anatomical site, tissue involved and nature of condition. The diagnosis allows the condition to be dealt with successfully, e.g., with surgery. Once these kinds of diagnoses have been eliminated as possibilities, however, we are left with non-surgical musculoskeletal problems such as common back pain.

A clinical method of examination, which Cyriax and others helped develop, can be applied for diagnosing such non-surgical problems. This method involves applying controlled physical stresses to the musculoskeletal system. Through knowledge of applied anatomy, it is often possible to apply a selective tension or stress to a specific muscle, joint or ligament. Usually this is done with one or two applications of tension or movement for each tissue being stressed. Based on a person's response to observed movement and to stress applied by the examiner, it may be possible to come to fairly reliable conclusions about the anatomical site and specific tissue that is the source of a person's symptoms. This approach seems to work reasonably well with areas of the body such as the shoulder or knee.

Except when neurological testing indicates that nerve damage exists from a herniated disc, diagnosing the specific tissue at fault in a case of back pain cannot be done very easily. In most cases of back pain, neurological damage is not evident. It may be possible to localize the general anatomical site of the problem, i.e., the moving parts of the spine. We may feel fairly sure that an activity-related problem exists. Nonetheless, the muscles, joints, ligaments, discs, etc., of the spine cannot be isolated easily from one another to perform selective tension testing. So in the case of a seemingly-simple back pain there exists an impasse for individual practitioners and individual patients looking to treat a specific tissue at fault

This impasse results from the view that "a lesion," a specific pathological tissue that is the source of pain, must always be found with certainty before successful treatment can be given for back pain. Although accepting this premise may sometimes have led to useful results, an absolutistic quest for "the lesion" may have blocked the path to more fruitful methods of therapy for many back pain patients.

Doctors and therapists and their patients can get hung up trying to find a traditional tissue diagnosis. The diagnosis can become more important than helping the patient. Some clinicians and researchers may latch onto a particular explanation of "the lesion" with a degree of certainty that is not actually warranted by the evidence. Others may throw up their hands in regard to the possibility of effective treatment other than watchful waiting. If they can't identify a specific lesion, they may call common everyday lower back pain "non-specific." Treatment of this 'non-specific' pain then often involves non-specific advice on posture and exercise. If you have back pain, you thereby are left in the dark, dependent upon passage of time.

The Primacy of Clinical Evidence

A specific tissue diagnosis involves some kind of theory, an inferred map or model that goes beyond what's directly observed. Such a diagnostic classification can give direction to the attempted treatment. However, in order to provide effective treatment when a particular diagnostic label remains in doubt, it may be desirable to deemphasize the label while not entirely neglecting it.

Cyriax's third principle was "All treatment must exert a beneficial effect on the lesion." How did he know that the treatment he provided had a beneficial effect? *He asked his patients!*

Cyriax, who used spinal manipulation (passive movements applied to the spine by doctor or therapist), advised systematic questioning and observation of the patient before and after every procedure. Despite his focus on diagnosis, clinical evidence—symptoms and observable posture and movement—had major importance for him.

Practitioners of a number of schools of posture-movement therapy have followed this line of thought. In spite of not clearly knowing the exact pathological source of many people's back problems, they often have been able to apply successful treatment by assessing its effects on the clinical evidence—how the patient feels and functions.

Australian physical therapist Geoffrey Maitland has pursued the insight of what he calls "the primacy of clinical evidence"[8] in a particularly detailed and systematic way:

Matching of the clinical findings to particular theories of anatomic, biomechanical, and pathological knowledge, so as to attach a particular "label" to the patient's condition, may not always be appropriate. Therapists must remain open-minded so that as treatment progresses, the patient is reassesssed in relation to the evolution of the condition and the responses to treatment.[9]

While this may seem like 'common sense', this approach to thinking, which Maitland has refined to an art, requires subtlety and skill and is not necessarily common.

Some steps in Maitland's concept of therapy can be useful to anyone treating back pain (including you when you seek to help yourself). These steps include:

1. Having assessed the effect of a patient's disorder [description of symptoms and observation of movements], to perform a single treatment technique

2. To take careful note of what happens during the performance of the technique

3. Having completed the technique, to assess the effect of the technique on the patient's symptoms including movements

4. Having assessed steps 2 and 3, and taken into account the available theoretical knowledge, to plan the next treatment approach and repeat the cycle from step 1 again[10]

Maitland has also emphasized that "the initial application of a technique must be gentle." These steps apply the scientific approach to problem-solving discussed in Chapter 1.

Mechanical Diagnosis and Therapy

The emphasis on clinical evidence has been taken a step further by physical therapist Robin McKenzie. McKenzie has created a unique system of mechanical (activity-related) diagnosis and therapy. Rather than focusing on discovering a specific tissue lesion, McKenzie's system focuses on the second element of diagnosis that Laslett mentioned, the nature of the condition.

Based on the effect of positions and movements on the patient's symptoms and movements, McKenzie has shown some ways to distinguish mechanical (activity-related) from non-mechanical back problems. He also has formulated several different categories of activity-related problems based on a person's symptoms and posture-movement patterns.

> The McKenzie approach is a system of assessment and therapeutics based on the recognition of patterns of mechanical and symptomatic responses to the stimuli of loading (applying forces to) the spine. This recognition is derived from historical information related by the patient as well as clinical findings that compare mechanical and symptomatic responses before, during, and after (1) singular movements, (2) repetitive movements, and (3) sustained positionings.[11]

What makes McKenzie's approach to diagnosis unique is its primary use of a person's own movements and positions rather than passive movements applied by a therapist. Treatment flows clearly from this method of testing. Because it starts with a person's own self-generated positions and movements, it encourages self-care.

McKenzie has promoted the use of repeated movement and sustained position testing.[12] These examination procedures are getting used increasingly often by spinal care practitioners of all types. What are they and how do they work?

During daily activities, your musculoskeletal system undergoes forces (loads) that involve varying amounts and directions of push or pull on the body. Mechanical (activity-related) pain is pain that can be produced, change location, increase, decrease or disappear as a result of these forces created by different positions and movements.

Think of the mechanical forces that affect your spine in the course of your normal daily activities. You may sit in front of a computer for an hour or more, with your lower back in a flexed position for most of that period of time. This involves a sustained position of asymmetrical force on your spine.

You may work in your garden and repeatedly bend, reach and lift. These repeated movements involve repetitive forces in one or a few directions. If you have back pain, *where* in your body you feel pain, *when* you feel it and *how easily or with what difficulty* you can move in various directions may very much depend on these kinds of 'normal' (though not necessarily beneficial) daily sustained positions and repeated movements.

The forces brought to bear on your spine from the one or two movements of a standard spinal examination cannot begin to simulate the forces that occur in your everyday activities. If the practitioner only observes one or two movements, how can he provide you with the specific, detailed and individualized advice you need to feel better as fast and completely as possible? He can't! Testing with repeated active movements and sustained positions creates forces on the structures of your spine in a way that comes closer to simulating the forces that occur with everyday activities.[13] By means of these forms of testing, a skilled practitioner can discover the particular effects of various positions and movements on your condition.

Your symptoms may include pain, tingling, pins and needles, and numbness that you can feel and report. Mechanical effects may include normal movement, movements limited by a certain amount or in a particular pattern, excessive movement, and/or distorted positions that you and the practitioner can observe.

A Repeated Movement examination includes having you actively move to *end range* (as far as your joints will go in each direction tested). The movements are done to your tolerance and only as many times as necessary to gain information about their effect on your symptoms and ability to move (ten times will often suffice). They are never done to the point of further injury. The basic movements for lower back testing include flexing and extending the back in the standing and lying positions, as well as other manuevers.

A practitioner using this method of examination will have already taken a thorough history. He will assess your sitting and standing posture. Then he will ask you to move once or twice through each of the test movements, similar to what is done in a standard back evaluation. This allows him to assess your range of voluntary movement in each direction.

Then he will ask you to describe the exact location and quality of your symptoms. You will repeat each movement and report on the location and quality of your symptoms both *during* and *at the end range* of a repeated series of movements. At the end of this repeated series you will report on your symptoms, their location and whether they seem better or worse. You may also be asked to assume one or more static positions to determine their effects on you.

This kind of examination provides a safe and controlled way to simulate the types of forces that you experience in your everyday activities. Carefully monitoring your symptoms and movement allows you and the practitioner to establish, with greater assurance, whether you do or do not have an activity-related (mechanical) problem.

If you do have a mechanical problem, it is possible to determine the specific nature of that problem in terms of the effects of positions and movements on your symptoms. As a result, you can receive an individualized program of treatment based on those *movements and positions that ease your symptoms.*

Using this approach does not require definitely knowing the exact anatomical source of the problem in order to resolve it. Even if the exact spinal tissue affected remains in doubt, a detailed examination using repeated movements and sustained positions can provide the information you need in order to have a beneficial effect on your symptoms.

The examination is based on your own active movements. In this way you have an opportunity from the start to find out how you can ease your symptoms through your own efforts. Your pain becomes a controlled variable. The practitioner works with you by guiding and coaching you through this process, which emphasizes self-care.

McKenzie's system, which he calls "mechanical diagnosis and therapy," starts with self-administered treatment. This is often sufficient to deal with problems and guarantees that patients have had the opportunity to learn how to deal with their own symptoms independently.

Rather than viewing exercises (self-applied movements) and manipulation (passively applied movements) as entirely separate categories of treatment, they can be viewed together on a continuum. Self-administered treatment may sometimes prove inadequate, even when it helps somewhat. A person may be moving in the right direction but not generating enough force to remain improved. At this point, therapist-generated forces (spinal manipulative therapy) can be used.

In this case, the results of repeated movement/sustained position testing and of the client's own efforts indicate in which direction to move the spine. Starting with the least amount of force, the therapist can apply pressure at the indicated level in the indicated direction. The therapist continually monitors the person's response. Using this approach, the therapist can safely increase the amount of force as needed. The purpose of this is to make self-treatment effective again.

Conclusion

In this chapter, I have indicated when you need to go to a medical doctor for diagnosis. Getting assurance that you do not have a serious medical problem is important. Once you have been told that you have mechanical (activity-related) back pain—what I call posture-movement-related pain—what do you do about it? Further diagnosis seems essential. But what kind of diagnosis?

When possible, finding "the lesion" can help. However, beyond a certain point, it often appears fruitless to search for a definitive diagnosis about the specific anatomical tissue at fault. When that is not possible with any degree of certainty, you still can get beneficial therapy.

Various therapy approaches use clinical evidence, changes in your symptoms and posture-movement patterns, to guide activity-related treatment. Because of the detailed attention to observing and describing what happens, this is different than just saying "it works."

I have described McKenzie's system of mechanical diagnosis and therapy as one example of this kind of approach. This system uses a person's own positions and movements to distinguish activity-related (mechanical) problems from non-activity-related ones. It also provides a way to distinguish different types of activity-related problems, allowing for a more specific posture-movement-based diagnosis. Self-treatment using a person's own posture and movement follows from this. Having been certified in this approach, I have found it useful in developing my own way of practicing posture-movement therapy—with due modesty, every practitioner develops his or her own way of practicing.

McKenzie's approach and the other approaches discussed in this chapter provide examples of some specific and effective 'maps' (models) for dealing with "non-specific" back pain. I have little doubt that other useful approaches exist or can be developed. I accept what science philosopher John Ziman wrote:

> [t]here is no simple "scientific" map of reality—or if there were, it would be much too complicated and unwieldy to be grasped or used by anyone. But there are many different maps of reality, from a variety of scientific viewpoints.[14]

In the following chapter, I present my own model of activity-related back pain that makes use of McKenzie's and others' approaches and which places them in a broader context. This map will provide the basis for my recommendations about what you can do now for your back pain.

Chapter 9

The Circles of Pain and Recovery

Previous chapters have explored the anatomy and physiology of the spine, the processes involved in experiencing pain and those by which we act to control our experience. The last chapter looked at the general process of getting a diagnosis. In this chapter, I will put together these factors into a posture-movement model to explain how activity-related back pain starts, gets perpetuated and then resolved.[1]

A Biopsychosocial Approach to Back Pain

Many researchers in the area of back pain show an increasing interest in the role of psychosocial factors in the origin, continuation of and treatment of back pain. In what has been called the "biopsychosocial" approach by Gordon Waddell, mechanical, psychological and social factors work together.[2] The posture-movement model presented in this chapter represents such a biopsychosocial approach, with the various factors working together in interacting and 'circular' negative feedback loops.

Because human behavior is purposeful, how you evaluate your back problem (what you believe and feel about it) can make a great difference in how you cope with it. This may ongoingly affect and be affected by how much pain you feel, how distressed you feel because of the pain, how disabled you may become as a result, and what you do to get better. This may all affect and be affected by the social environment of your family, work, health care practitioners, and the larger society.

The most accurate way to consider the biological (including activity-related), psychological and social factors always present in back pain is not to treat them as if they were en-

tirely separate and isolated. Indeed, adequate posture-movement-related evaluation reveals part of the biological aspect
of the problem in a way that can also help build a positive psychosocial climate for the person experiencing back pain and
disability.

The Circle of Injury and Pain

Figure 9.1 on the next page shows the first half of my posture-movement model. It shows important stages (italicized
in the text) in the process of initially responding to injury and
pain. The key below lists and briefly defines these stages. Unfortunately, the useful process of initial response to injury can
sometimes lead to a self-perpetuating vicious circle of disuse
and pain, which I will explain in the section following this one.

Key to Figure 9.1

Environment: As organisms-as-wholes-in-environments
we transact with objects and processes such as air, food,
gravity, etc.; other organisms (microbes, cats, dogs, etc.);
other people and the resulting social-cultural processes
(language, beliefs, etc.). The environment of each
individual's nervous system also includes what goes on inside and on the skin. "The animal does not merely adapt
to the environment, but also constantly adapts the environment to itself."[3]

Initial Injury: Visible or microscopic disruption or damage to soft tissues of body (muscle, joint, disc, ligaments,
etc.) through undue application of force.

Inflammation: Sequel to injury characterized by swelling,
redness, heat and pain. May also result from infection and
from certain inflammatory diseases.

Sensory Impact: Immediate information (feedback) about
internal and external environments.

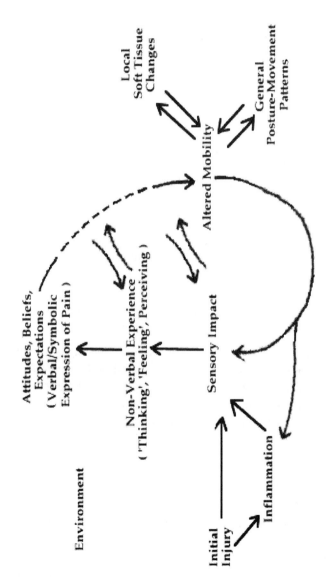

Figure 9.1 – The Potentially Vicious Circle of Pain and Disuse

Non-Verbal Experience: Higher-level nervous system processes of which organism has awareness. Shared by animals and humans. Involves 'thinking', 'feeling', perceiving without words.

Attitudes, Beliefs, Expectations: 'Thinking', 'feeling', perceiving expressed and elaborated in words and other symbols. Through complex, circular feedback mechanisms, these are both influenced by and influence ongoing *Sensory Impacts* and *Non-Verbal Experiences*.

Altered Mobility: Efforts affected by and further affecting our experience of injury and/or pain. Includes withdrawal from external source of damage (considered trivial) and more important stage of guarding (protective holding) of painful area.

General Posture-Movement Patterns: Global organism-as-a-whole changes of posture and movement related to *Altered Mobility*. Posture-movement patterns can develop as a response to local changes in muscles and joints following injury, inflammation and healing. They may also be based on imitation of others, on emotional factors, e.g. slump of depression, and may become habitual.

Local Soft Tissue Changes: Local tissue changes in joints, ligaments, discs, muscles, etc., related to *Altered Mobility* following injury, inflammation and healing of these tissues. May also occur as consequence of continuing guarding and immobility and as a result of poor *General Posture-Movement Patterns*.

An *initial injury* occurs. As the result of some visible trauma, bone, muscle, joint capsules, ligaments, discs, nerves and other tissues can suffer. Forces strong enough to bruise, stretch, tear or compress one or more of these tissues of the spine may cause immediate pain from the damaging stress.

Physiology texts traditionally have focused on the importance of a sudden reflex-like withdrawing from the source of damage at the time of this *sensory impact*. This can be represented in the diagram by the arrows leading from *sensory impact* to *altered mobility* and back to *sensory impact*, a relatively simple lower-level feedback loop. However, pain researcher Patrick Wall considers this kind of reaction trivial and rather over-emphasized in people's efforts to understand human responses to pain.[4]

Following the immediate damage, sensory nerves in the area respond by releasing chemicals that dilate local blood vessels. These can also stimulate pain. In addition, products from the broken cells of damaged tissues and the enzymes that break down these products both provide chemical irritants that can trigger additional pain.[5]

Thus begins the process of *inflammation* and its familiar signs of swelling, redness, heat and pain. In a peripheral injury, such as a sprained wrist or ankle, we can observe this more easily than in a back injury. The swelling walls off and isolates the area of injury as fluids from the dilated blood vessels move into the tissue spaces. White blood cells also move into the area to clear up the damaged tissue.

Inflammation provides the basis for repair of damaged tissues. Cells called fibroblasts begin the process of forming new connective tissue. New blood vessels and nerve fibers may also grow. This process of healing creates a scar which knits together the broken elements. Both the swelling and the cellular cleanup and healing operations may provide chemical sources of inflammatory pain.[6]

This inflammatory response can occur not only with injury but also in cases of inflammatory illnesses, such as rheumatoid arthritis. Such illnesses involve the inappropriate activation of an inflammatory response due to some malfunctioning of the immune system. The chemical by-products produced during such an episode can also result in tissue destruction. Posture-movement related problems may exist once such an active epsode has passed.

The sensory impact of injury and inflammation continues ongoingly. The upward-directed arrows from *sensory impact* to *non-verbal experience* to *attitudes, beliefs, expectations* represent various levels of the nervous system experience of pain illustrated in Chapter 6, Figure 6.1. As you can perhaps see more clearly now, the sensory impact and non-verbal experience steps also represent the input side of a complex negative feedback control hierarchy, as described in Chapter 7.

A downwardly-directed arrow moves from *attitudes, beliefs, expectations* towards *altered mobility.* This arrow has breaks in it to indicate that the influence of the higher level of beliefs, expectations, etc., is not direct. Rather, as indicated in the chapter on control theory, the outputs of higher levels exert their influence on lower levels by providing internal standards (reference signals) which ultimately affect the actions of the organism.

The arrows pointing in towards and then out from lower levels indicate that *beliefs*, etc., affect *non-verbal experience*; *beliefs* and *non-verbal experience* in turn influence the level of *sensory impact.* The full extent of these influences includes internal changes in the nervous system (remember the gate theory) and hormonal and immune system changes, as well as observable efforts that you make. All of these occur within an *environment*, both 'physical' and 'social', which influences and in turn is influenced by what you do.

Your pain may tend to powerfully capture your attention; yet your immediate environment, other concerns that you attend to, the meanings you give to the situation, your beliefs and expectations (both personal and culturally-derived) may all have very real effects on your ongoing experience and on your physiology. This provides the basis for understanding the beneficial (placebo) or harmful (nocebo) effects of suggestions and expectations.[7]

Psychiatrist and neurobiologist J. Allan Hobson writes:
...consciousness is causal, and in a very material way....since subjectivity is itself a brain [nervous system] function, it very naturally can redirect its own energy from one neural region to another.[8]

Let's return to what happens following an injury. You can trace the arrows directed out and to the side from *non-verbal experience* and from *sensory impact* and follow their path to *altered mobility.* These arrows suggest the organism-as-a-whole-in-an-environment process related to posture and movement that takes place once damage has occurred and inflammation has set in.

The process of *altered mobility* following injury involves guarding, reducing the amount of local movement in the damaged area to allow the repair process to adequately take place. As Wall describes it:

> All of us have minor accidents several times a year, often so minor that we may forget them, but, during the recovery time, we guard the damaged area, protect it, and move it as little as possible. That motor behavior, which is the opposite of the sudden brief withdrawal, is crucial for recovery because the area of damage cannot complete the inflammatory and recovery processes if it is moving and under pressure.[9]

Guarding a damaged area after an injury constitutes a healthy and necessary process. It completes a negative feedback loop by providing the means for controlling the ongoing *sensory impact* and thus reducing the *non-verbal experience* of pain. It allows the process of recovery to proceed without further aggravation. Wall points out the disastrous consequences of minor injuries for those people who have a rare condition called congenital analgesia. These people do not experience pain and subsequently do not guard their movements, thus continuing to damage their joints, increase inflammation, etc.[10]

Guarding actions involve the organism-as-a-whole. To indicate this, an arrow points down and to the right from *altered movement* towards *general posture-movement patterns.* This outward-pointing arrow and the reverse arrow represent global changes in posture and movement related to localized altered mobility following injury. Wall notes:

> Joints are splinted by the highly unusual, steady, simultaneous contractions of all of the muscles that can move the joint...Dogs are a wonderful example of the widespread readjustment of muscles produced by a small injury to one foot. They switch effortlessly to a three-legged gait with one foot steadily flexed. This requires an instant reorganization of all the leg and body muscles. And so it does with us.[11]

Changes in *general posture-movement patterns* can occur by means of feedback loops of conscious and unconscious behavior that control potentially painful perceptions.

These posture-movement patterns are associated with other organism-as-a-whole changes involving the autonomic nervous system, which regulates the hormone-secreting glands, the heart muscle and the smooth muscles of the blood vessels, gut and other internal organs. Under calm conditions, there exists a balance between the parasympathetic and the sympathetic parts of this system. The parasympathetic system generally slows heart rate, increases circulation to the limbs and surface of the body, and aids the digestion of food. The sympathetic system, the "fright, fight, flight" component, raises the heart rate, shifts circulation to the muscles and body core, and reduces digestion and movements in the gut. When you experience pain, your autonomic balance will tip towards this sympathetic response of "fright and flight."[12]

Another arrow from *altered mobility* points up and to the right towards *local soft tissue changes.* Here we change the scale of interest from general posture-movement patterns to a much more narrow focus on particular muscle, joint, and other tissue changes. As mentioned in the previous chapter, various practitioners have found it difficult to agree on diagnosing the particular tissue (muscle, joint, disc, etc.) responsible for common back pain. Nonetheless, injury and the processes of inflammation and healing (via scar tissue formation) undoubtedly can occur in any of these tissues. Through the kind of testing discussed in the previous chapter, movement patterns and pain responses can help to determine what tissue might be affected. More importantly, such testing can help determine the appropriateness of any particular posture-movement strategy to help restore normal function.

The Vicious Circle of Disuse and Pain

Immediately after injury, inflammation may predominate. and you may feel pain all of the time. With inflammation pain, what McKenzie calls "chemical pain,"[13] reducing your movement has some usefulness. However, even here some ways of reducing movement, i.e., staying as relaxed as possible while maintaining neutral spinal postures, may be better than "a body fixed in an overall pain posture."[14]

Once an injury has occurred and healing has taken place, pain and altered mobility may continue past the point where they serve much useful purpose. Some pains may get incorrectly interpreted as meaning further damage. This leads to continued guarding of posture and movement to avoid the pains which get interpreted as more damage and lead to more guarding, etc. You can trace the circle in Figure 9.1 that goes around and around in this way.

Wall describes this circle of disuse, pain and more disuse as follows:

> Muscles are in steady contraction and, as time goes by, some muscles grow while joints and tendons deteriorate because [the] frozen posture sets off local changes....the problem is to override a natural defence mechanism that has a protective role in brief emergencies but becomes maladaptive when prolonged....movement that produces pain does not necessarily increase the injury...lack of movement that seems at first to prevent pain eventually acts to prolong pain.[15]

Many practitioners in the posture-movement field have pointed out that hurt does not necessarily equal harm. The existence of pain does not necessarily mean the existence of damage. Understanding the kinds of *Soft Tissue Changes* that can occur after injury can help you to understand and better deal with these not necessarily harmful pains.

Soft Tissue Changes

Changes in the soft tissues, e.g., muscles, joints, etc., resulting in limited movement, have been called "contractures" by physical therapy researchers Cummings, Crutchfield and Barnes.[16] They group soft tissue contractures into three main categories:

1. The formation of adhesions in the muscles, tendons, joint capsules, ligaments, etc., as a result of injury and scar tissue formation; [17]

2. Adaptive shortening in uninjured muscles and skin that occurs as a result of altered mobility and guarding; [18]

3. Joint displacements that involve restriction of movement "due to malpositioning of the articular surfaces of the joint."[19]

Let's look first at how adhesions get formed. As healing happens, connective tissue cells begin producing new fibers that will 'fill in' with new connective tissue whatever tissue has been damaged. This process, called scarring, may begin several days after a back injury and can continue for several weeks until the new tissue gets layed down. While this happens, too much movement, especially vigorous end range movement in the wrong direction, may interfere with the process and interrupt connective tissue formation.

At some point, however, scar tissue gets formed and will begin to mature. At this stage, inadequate movement will result in an adhesion, a shortened, stiffened area, painful at its restricted end range. McKenzie calls this kind of condition a "dysfunction syndrome." [20] Movement testing can help to determine if this kind of situation exists.

Pain in this case is not something to avoid. Restricted motion associated with pain that you feel intermittently at end range and which doesn't worsen with repetitions means that tightened structures are getting stretched. No damage occurs. In fact, you must feel that type of tolerable 'stretch pain' for the movement to do any good. While a newly-formed scar matures, one can apply enough beneficial stress to it through movement so that it will reform in a strong, lengthened, unrestricted and painless way.

Such "dysfunctions" do not result only from direct injury, since a second type of contracture, "adaptive shortening," can affect even uninjured muscles and skin. These tissues can become adaptively shortened over time if they do not have adequate movement. Muscles, for example, can change their length, sometimes quite quickly, if they are constantly splinting a painful joint or when they otherwise become overworked by constant contraction and fatigue. [21]

A third kind of *soft tissue change* or contracture, "joint displacement," can also contribute to a circle of disuse and pain. This is not a dislocated joint. Rather, a change occurs in the relationship between the articulating surfaces of a joint so that normal movement is restricted. This seems similar to what McKenzie calls the "derangement syndrome." [22]

If you have this kind of back problem, you may feel constant pain. However, unlike the pain associated with inflammation, symptoms will vary with the time of day and with different positions and movements. You may or may not be fixed in a position of deformity. What is going on here?

According to Cummings, et al.:

> ...at a normal joint...bone B moves around bone A. The
> articulating surfaces remain in contact and the looseness
> of the capsule and ligaments allow the excursion [normal

movement] to take place...[With a joint displacement] bone B for some reason is displaced on bone A in the starting position. You will find that it will not be possible for bone B to move all the way around bone A. The range-of-motion will be limited. This limitation may be caused by intricacies of the articulating surfaces such as configurational mismatches, curves of the articulating surfaces, or bits of meniscus [cartilage pads], which may cause the joint to lock....Another possible cause of joint limitation by displacement is reflex inhibition of muscle action.[23]

Following the work of orthopedic physician James Cyriax, McKenzie has argued that this kind of problem in the back most often results from changes within the disc. According to this disc model of joint "derangement," small reversible shifts of material within the disc can occur that exert constant mechanical stress upon pain-sensitive structures of the spine.

As previously noted in Chapter 5, the disc consists of a fibrous outer wall and a gel-like inner portion. With normal aging, so-called "degenerative" changes, such as cracks and fissures, can occur within the structure of the disc. As the result of trauma or as a result of abnormal asymmetrical stresses — such as poor and prolonged sitting and frequent and prolonged flexion of the spine — displacement of material can occur within the joint.[24]

When this occurs, something within the disc, perhaps some of the gel material, has moved from its normal position inside the joint. This distorted material may not then change position as quickly as necessary when further movement requires such change. Instead, pain and loss of movement occurs as the joint and surrounding tissues are placed under abnormal stress. Severe changes in *general posture-movement patterns* may occur, visible as postural deformities, as part of a strategy to reduce the resulting pain.

This "derangement process" takes time to occur—the result, over time, of undesirable repeated movements or prolonged positioning. It will usually take time and the application of the proper repeated movements and sustained positions to make things right again.

Surgeons and other physicians are familiar with the extreme state of this disorder. With a herniated disc, extruded material presses into the surrounding tissue spaces, causing nerve irritation and injury.

Under these circumstances, especially when it first occurs, positions and movements will probably not have much of an effect in reducing symptoms. Time will be needed for the surrounding tissues to accommodate to the extruded material, which may also shrink over time. Surgery, however, sometimes may be a good option here.

Short of this extreme, when the wall containing the gel contents of the disc seems intact, it often is possible to reduce internal disc derangements . Posture-movement therapy apparently can then change the shape and location of displaced material and restore normal relations within the spinal structures.

Movement testing can indicate which movements and positions will reduce or abolish symptoms, or change where symptoms are felt. With derangements, this change in where symptoms are felt seems especially notable.[25]

Clinicians have observed for years that the pain resulting from a back injury often starts in or near the middle of the back. As it worsens it can either spread out or shift away from the spine and into one or the other buttock or leg. McKenzie calls this *peripheralization*, since symptoms have moved out to the periphery of the body.

It has become more apparent in recent years that as symptoms improve they may decrease at, or move away from, the periphery and move closer to the center of the spine. For example, in the case of Paul, about whom I talked in Chapter 3, the pain that he felt going into his leg and calf reduced and disappeared as his symptoms and ability to move improved. Concurrently, he noticed more symptoms near the center of his back for awhile. McKenzie uses the term *centralization* for this phenomenon of pain decreasing or shifting out of the periphery and moving closer to the center. Centralization provides a consistently reliable guide for effective treatment.[26]

Peripheralization and centralization may correspond respectively to increased and decreased joint displacement due to distortion and disruption within a disc. Many physical therapists, physicians and chiropractors still do not accept the model of disc derangement as explained above. Nonetheless, a significant amount of research provides evidence in its favor.[27] Treatment based on this model works effectively much of the time.

Posture-Movement Patterns & the Vicious Circle

General posture-movement patterns provide ways of dealing with immediate injury and subsequent inflammation. As healing proceeds, contractures develop in muscles and joints. As a result, posture-movement patterns also develop as coping strategies for dealing with these soft tissue changes. As discussed in Chapter 4, these patterns can also develop through imitation of others, through ongoing emotional factors, e.g., the slump of depression, and also as default habits in the course of your activities of daily living.

Cyriax's assumption that "All pain arises from a lesion" (mentioned in Chapter 8) is not correct. Sometimes your posture-movement patterns may cause pain in the absence of injury or any joint or muscle problems. McKenzie uses the example of the "bent finger."[28] Take one of your fingers and bend it backwards with a finger of the other hand. Bend it back as far as you can. Make it hurt! Now relax your finger.

Do you have something wrong with your finger? If you answered no, that doesn't mean that your pain is 'just in your head' (whatever that means!). When you bent your finger back, you didn't damage anything. However, the pain presumably provided some warning of impending damage that might occur if you continued to stress the ligaments, joints, etc., of your finger.

Some people experience back pain after long periods of slumped sitting or standing. When tested, they appear painfree and have full spinal mobility. McKenzie calls this kind of pain the "postural syndrome," because a movement examination yields normal results and symptoms only appear with sustained bad postures.[29] In this case, back pain, just like the bent finger, doesn't necessarily indicate damage. Rather, the pain seems to provide a warning signal. When an individual who has this kind of condition begins to guard and restrict movement because of the pain he experiences, he does exactly the opposite of what he needs to do, which is to sit less and become more active.

If poor posture-movement habits continue long enough, they may lead to soft tissue contractures due to adaptive shortening. Micro-trauma and inflammation also may become factors here.

Thinking in Other Categories

The pathways of circular causation and the multiple soft tissue changes that can happen together at one time guarantee that a vicious circle can sometimes seem like a confusing maze. In addition to what I've already discussed here, Laslett and van Wijman have listed a number of types of diagnoses that may also be involved in a circle of disuse and back pain:

sacro-iliac joint problems, mechanical instability, facet joint problems, spinal stenosis and psychologically-based illness behavior.[30]

Whatever the problem, usually more than one tissue gets affected when someone develops spinal soft tissue changes. Even those areas that did not get directly injured may feel tight and uncomfortable. Very likely muscles, joints, discs, ligaments, etc., all need to have normal movement restored once an acute injury has occured. Muscles will need to recover the strength and endurance through their full range that they may have lost when normal movements could not occur.

Recovery of normal movement seems necessary because continuing soft tissue changes and their concurrent posture-movement patterns increase the likelihood of future problems. Abnormally shortened scar tissue or adaptively shortened muscles do not have the strength or resiliency of normal tissues. They can more easily get pulled, overstretched, and reinjured during normal activities.

Other complicating factors exist as well. For example, various pain syndromes associated with nerve damage appear to have a part to play in the back-related pain problems experienced by some people. Injury to a spinal nerve may result in a vicious circle because of an increase in sensitivity to normal stimulation after the initial damage has resolved.

In the case of chronic back pain, chronic inflammation may provide another complicating factor. This may include originally injured tissues and secondary areas affected by a circle of pain and immobility.[31]

Psychogenic Pain

One category noted above, "psychologically-based illness behavior," deserves further discussion. If done at all, making this diagnosis requires extreme caution since it often represents a mistaken attempt to separate the 'body' (bio) from the 'mind' (psychosocial).

In understanding the circle of back pain and disuse, psychosocial factors always need to be considered. Nonetheless, probably only a very few people have what could be called purely psychosocial 'back pain' and actually fake back problems (malinger). In addition, although some people with back pain may dramatize or magnify it in order to gain attention, compensation, relief from responsibilties, etc., it is not clear that this involves more than a small number of individuals.

In Chapter 6, I briefly mentioned the related notion of *psychogenic pain*. Those who apply this diagnosis consider most back pain to have a primary psychological origin. John Sarno, M.D., a physical medicine (rehabilitation) specialist, advocates this view. Sarno contends that internal conflicts, anxieties, etc., often get translated directly into muscle tension in the back which then causes pain. He believes that this accounts for a large proportion of back problems.[32]

According to Sarno, the best treatment for such a problem consists of convincing the patient that his symptoms are due to psychological conflicts. Accepting this 'diagnosis' often seems sufficient to solve the problem, although he does recommend providing some level of counseling at times.

With this approach, physical therapy may serve as an adjunct to help promote general mobility. However, for the most part, patients are advised to forget about special exercises, body mechanics, etc., to stop worrying about pain, and to simply return to normal activity.

Sarno's view of psychogenic back pain has some merit in that it points to the importance of attitudes, anxiety and guarding in perpetuating back problems. Quite likely, some of his successes have been with individuals who had became so fearful about reinjuring themselves that their self-imposed guarding became a major part of their ongoing disability. In some of these cases, anxiety reduction leading to normal, unguarded movement may have sufficed to correct minor soft tissue contractures.

However, sometimes a change in attitude, although necessary, may not in itself be sufficient to get better. I have worked with a number of people who, prior to seeing me, attempted to exert their 'minds' over their back problems. They felt like failures when they did not succeed in getting rid of their 'psychologically-caused' pain. This obviously didn't help their ability to cope.

Advocates of the psychogenic approach to back pain have oversimplified the relations among emotional factors, movement and pain. They also underestimate the importance of the kinds of soft tissue changes in the joints and muscles that I've discussed so far. As you can see in the posture-movement model presented in this chapter, emotional factors, soft tissue changes and postural factors all work together to perpetuate a circle of pain and disuse.

Faulty Effort

A simple, linear relation between so-called psychological factors and pain does not exist. Neither does there exist a simple linear relation between mechanical joint problems and pain. Exclusively psychological approaches (as these are usually understood) or those that focus only on joint and muscle mechanics cannot provide a comprehensive approach for dealing with back pain.

The circular causal, biopsychosocial model presented here does provide the basis for such an approach. This model is supported by the work of Whatmore and Kohli on faulty effort, which they call "dysponesis":

> ... "dys" meaning bad, faulty, or wrong, and "ponos" meaning effort, work, or energy. The term [dysponesis] thus identifies the basic nature of the condition, namely, a physiopathological state made up of errors in energy expenditure within the nervous system...If a patient's symp-

toms have their origin in dysponesis but he is treated only for structural disease or only to resolve psychological problems, results will be disappointing, for dysponesis is a neurophysiological response pattern that will survive these forms of treatment.[33]

The initial guarding (what Whatmore and Kohli call a "bracing effort") in the first stages of musculoskeletal injury may serve as an appropriate way for dealing with that situation. When bracing, associated with increased sympathetic activation, becomes an ongoing response to any experience of discomfort with movement (even if such movement may ultimately prove beneficial) than the guarding has become inappropriate, a faulty effort.

Faulty effort may also initiate a back problem in the absence of any apparent injury. Bracing and also the inappropriate body mechanics involved in slumping and poor posture (which can also be considered a form of faulty effort) may lead first to warning pains in muscles and joints (McKenzie's posture syndrome) and then microtrauma and inflammation that can begin a circle of symptoms. It will also add additional stress to any existing problems in the muscles and joints.

Whatmore and Kohli suggest that faulty effort can be measured through the use of biofeedback machines which show the electrical activity associated with muscular effort. They suggest the use of biofeedback training to recognize, reduce and eliminate faulty efforts.

However, you don't necessarily need a machine to observe the signs of what F. M. Alexander called "undue effort": held breath, clenched jaw, tensed muscles, dilated pupils, cold, sweaty palms and feet, etc. Many methods exist that may help you reduce faulty effort, including study of the Alexander Technique, other forms of posture-movement education, hypnosis and relaxation methods, among others.

Chronic Pain

If you have had chronic back pain, you have been looping around a circle of pain and disuse for months or years. You may have given up hope.

Depression, anger and fear can act like lenses that magnify and concentrate pain and guarding. You can deal with these emotions successfully with some combination of medication and counseling. In the next section, I will discuss more about the importance of your attitude in coping with back pain.

The neurological processing of pain can also sometimes get altered in chronic pain situations. Specific medications and other treatments exist that work very effectively with specific types of pain. There is a growing medical specialty of pain management. If you have an ongoing pain problem, you may do well to consider getting a referral to a medical doctor credentialed in this field.

When more health care practitioners begin to use and not simply talk about the biopsychosocial approach to back problems, it will be easier for people with chronic pain to receive a comprehensive approach to their problems that includes the best that education, medicine, physical therapy and psychology presently have to offer.

The Vital Circle of Recovery

On the following page, Figure 9.2 shows the stages involved in entering a vital circle of pain control and recovery. The diagram shows that getting out of the vicious circle of disuse may start in a number of interrelated ways. Remember that as an organism-as-a-whole-in-an-environment, you constitute a complicated multi-dimensional system. Even one small positive change can begin to make a difference to the whole system since "we can never do merely one thing."[34]

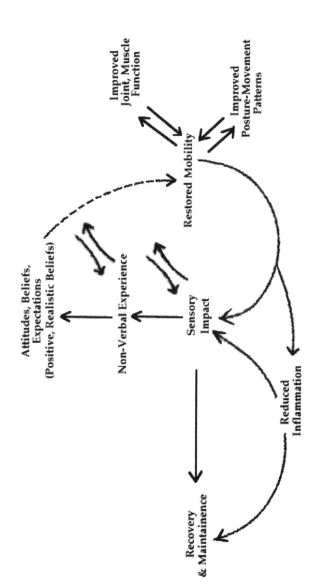

Figure 9.2 – The Vital Circle of Recovery

For example, if you have soft tissue changes you may on your own or with assistance begin to improve joint and muscle function with particular positions and movements. You can begin to distinguish hurts that harm from hurts that don't—a point I will elaborate in the next chapter. Apart from specific effects on soft tissues, gentle movement also can have important pain-reducing effects, according to the Gate Theory discussed in Chapter 6. Improving your posture-movement habits can also have an important effect in controlling pain by reducing faulty effort and subsequent irritation and inflammation in muscles and joints. You can find more details about how to improve your posture-movement habits in Section IV of this book.

Although it can help a great deal, working on the mechanical aspects of your problems may not be sufficient to deal with your negative beliefs and emotions. If you have become overwhelmed by pain, anxiety, depression, etc., there are medications that can help. Coaching, counseling or psychotherapy may also have special importance in helping you move out of the disabling circle of pain, fear, posture-movement limitations and more pain.

Ultimately, it's up to you. Perhaps the most important thing you can do is to recognize the possibility of doing better. Changing your attitude towards your back problem will make other parts of the vital circle roll more steadily towards recovery.

When appropriate, I tell people about the ABCs of emotional self-care developed by psychologist Albert Ellis, the founder of Rational Emotive Behavior Therapy (REBT). I refer them to books and, if needed, to a qualified REBT-trained coach, counselor or therapist.

REBT is based, in part, on the ancient wisdom of the Stoic philosopher Epictetus, who wrote that "What disturbs people's minds is not events but their judgments on events." Ellis has built upon this to describe the ABCs of emotions. "A" stands for an Activating event, an occurence or situation with which we deal. "B" stands for Beliefs, the judgments that we make on events based on our experiences, expectations, assumptions and attitudes. "C" refers to the emotional Consequences which, Ellis posits, result from these beliefs.

The beliefs that often get us into emotional trouble are those that involve absolutistic demands on the way circumstances, other people and ourselves 'should' be. It may be appropriate at times to get mildly upset for more or less brief periods when things don't go as we prefer. However, the severe and ongoing emotional distress that we feel, even under the most dire circumstances, seems to result to a significant extent from our belief that things *must* go the way we absolutistically demand that they go.

Ellis suggests that you can learn to dispute your irrational beliefs about how things 'should' be by turning these absolutistic demands into liberating preferences. How does this relate to your back problem? It is not unlikely that you have been making yourself unnecessarily miserable about your problem. Since you are your own most enchanted listener, you can start now by listening to your own self-talk for absolutistic and unrealistic "musts," "shoulds," "always's," "nevers," "can'ts," etc.

As Ellis points out in his book *How To Stubbornly Refuse To Make Yourself Miserable About Anything, Yes Anything!*, it is important to practice

> ...distinguishing between appropriate concern, caution, vigilance and inappropriate anxiety, nervousness, and panic....Whenever you have strong negative feelings because unfortunate things are actually happening to you or you imagine that they might occur, see whether these feelings appropriately follow from your *wishes* and *desires* to have better things occur. Or are you creating them by go-

ing beyond your preferences and inventing powerful *shoulds, oughts, musts, demands, commands,* and *necessities*? If so, you are turning concern and caution into *over*concern, severe anxiety, and panic. Observe the real difference in your feelings![35]

Besides disputing your irrational demands about your problem, you can also remember that there is life beyond your back pain. In the search for solutions, you may have become so over-focused on your problem that back pain threatens to become your career. There is no need to wait until you're painfree before you shift your attention to wider goals and interests. Ellis advises to

try to become involved in a long-term purpose, goal, or interest in which you can remain truly absorbed. *Make* yourself a good, happy life by giving yourself something to live *for*. In that way you will distract yourself from serious woes and will help preserve your mental health.[36]

And while you are learning to stubbornly refuse to make yourself miserable about your back pain, cultivate your sense of humor! Remember that "Laughter is a tranquilizer with no side effects." [37]

In the next chapter, you will find specific guidelines on what to do to avoid and escape a vicious circle of pain so you can roll along a vital circle of pain control and recovery.

Chapter 10

Now What Do You Do?

Guidelines For Recovery

You can begin to use the posture-movement model presented in the previous chapter by contemplating Figure 9.1 and considering some of the ways that you may have gotten stuck in a circle of disuse and pain.

Then consider Figure 9.2, which suggests a number of overlapping and interconnected steps in the circle of recovery which have special importance for posture-movement therapy:

 • Develop positive, realistic beliefs about your problem.

 • Restore mobility, which includes reduction of unnecessary guarding.

 • Improve joint, muscle function (reduce specific soft tissue contractures).

 • Improve general posture-movement patterns.

The ways these steps overlap and interconnect have major importance. You can never merely do one thing. Improving one area will have reverberating effects on the others. This provides a reason for the variety of approaches that can work to help you control and recover from your back problem.

In this chapter, I present five general guidelines to help you to reduce your back pain symptoms and to circle towards recovery:

1. Make a secure start by getting medical help when needed.

2. Reduce unnecessary guarding (dysponesis) which may have reduced your mobility.

3. Index your symptoms.

4. Explore possibilities for extending your spine as you improve joint and muscle function and increase mobility.

5. Improve your posture-movement habits.

What particular things would you like to change? These can be specific joint or muscle problems that you have experienced, one or more aspects of your posture that you would like to improve, one or more activities that you have stopped or restricted and that you would like to feel more comfortable with, among other factors.

As you read this chapter, use the various guidelines to help you formulate some specific results that you would like to achieve and at least one thing you can do to help bring about each result. Remember that the more specifically you can state things, the more likely success. Find some way, no matter how small, to experience some success now. You can modify, add to and/or replace your goals and "to do" list as you proceed.

Make A Secure Start

Back pain can come from many sources. Although most of the time pain results from activity-related (posture-movement) stresses, you can make a secure start by ruling out any 'red flag' conditions which may, at least for now, militate against posture-movement therapy. You can do this by seeing a medical doctor as previously detailed in Chapter 8. You are encouraged to review that material if you have any questions about whether or not to consult a physician. Writing down your answers to the 'red flag' questions can be helpful.

Your physician most likely will not have the knowledge or time necessary to give you specific and individualized functional advice regarding your condition. However, he or she should be able to determine the likelihood of your having a mechanical disorder. Just knowing that you don't have a serious illness can reduce your anxiety and help you to cope better. Your medical doctor may be able to refer you to a health care practitioner who specializes in spinal rehabilitation. Your medical doctor can also advise you regarding anti-inflammatory and pain medication that may help you deal more effectively with this episode.

If you have already received a diagnosis for a chronic and/or recurring back problem, you may also benefit from getting medical advice if you feel depressed, have sleep problems and/or unremitting pain. Effective medications and treatment regimens exist. Family practitioners and internists are increasingly aware of the importance of pain management. If unable to provide such care him/herself, your physician should be able to refer you to a pain management clinic or to a specialist in this growing field.

Reduce Unnecessary Guarding

Soon after injury occurs, guarding (bracing) works as a useful way of controlling pain perceptions while the processes of healing can take place. At some point, sufficient healing will have occurred so that the need for normal movement can take precedence. Guarding may nonetheless continue even though it has become unnecessary. Even at earlier stages when some reduced movement seems appropriate, the 'wisdom' of the body may overdo things with excessive guarding efforts that take on a life of their own.

At these earlier stages of recovery from injury, unneeded bracing may impair further healing by preventing movements that would reduce swelling. At later stages, guarding may prevent the remodeling of adhesions if the normal stretch pains associated with this process are interpreted as damage. As explained earlier, excessive and prolonged guarding may also lead to further soft tissue contractures from adaptive shortening in the muscles and skin.

Application of the other guidelines for recovery can help to reduce unnecessary guarding. For example, sometimes a change in attitude and reduction in anxiety may be enough to reduce some guarding. That's one reason why it's important to get medical help initially. This may also explain some of the successes of psychogenic approaches to treatment.

It can also help if you understand your stage of recovery and the kind of movement-related problem you have. You can discover this through posture and movement testing by a qualified health professional. This can help you reduce fear and anxiety about those pains that may hurt but not harm. In the section on indexing pain, I'll review the different kinds of pain and what they signify in terms of desirable and undesirable movements for different kinds of soft tissue problems.

The section following that one will then guide you through a posture-movement sequence from Robin McKenzie's work. This progression of positions and movements, which emphasizes spinal extension (bending backwards), has often proved useful in reducing symptoms (including guarding) and restoring normal mobility.

Attention to your posture-movement habits can also make a great difference in reducing excessive guarding and in finding the appropriate amount of effort. I address this in Part IV, which follows this chapter.

In the remainder of this section, I'll discuss some ways that you can directly address the issue of unnecessary guarding (dysponesis).

Guarding and Breath

Sympathetic "fright, fight, flight" activation can accompany the guarding mode. Your breathing pattern may reflect this stressful emotional state. This pattern may involve rapid shallow breathing or breath holding. Simple observation of your breathing can help you to reduce this state and activate the parasympathetic side of your autonomic nervous system. This will promote general relaxation by reducing anxiety and excessive muscle tension.

Here are two simple breathing techniques that you can do anywhere. However, if you feel a great deal of discomfort they may work most effectively if you lie down in as comfortable a position as you can.

The first technique, called "the thirty-six breaths" is described by Alice Burmeister in her book, *The Touch of Healing*:

Begin by counting your exhalations. ("One, exhale, inhale. Two, exhale, inhale. Three, exhale, inhale." And so on.) Count until you have completed thirty-six breaths. If you lose count, you can start again. This can be done at one time or throughout the day, counting in four groups of nine. Allow your breathing to unfold naturally. In time, your breathing will automatically become deeper and more rhythmic.[1]

As you practice this method, notice the movements related to your breathing in your rib cage, your abdomen, your back and elsewhere. As you notice these naturally occurring movements, perhaps you can begin to allow them to occur more freely. Notice what effects this has on how you feel and on your ability to move and function.

Another breathing method that takes even less time to do comes from Dr. Kay Thompson, a dentist and psychologist who taught the following as a relaxation technique:

Press the tips of your index finger and your thumb together in a circle as you take a deep breath and hold it for a count of five. Let your breath out slowly as you release your thumb and index fingers and let them come apart (the finger tips serve as a cue for the change from tension to relaxation that you want to experience here). Then take another five relaxed breaths, counting your exhalations as in the previous method. Stay focused on your breath. Notice where you feel relaxed as a result of doing this. You can develop a relaxation habit by practicing this at least three times per day. Use it whenever you feel anxious or when you feel the need to release some tension.[2]

Guarding and Movement Sensation

Guarding efforts reduce movement which reduces sensation which in turn reduces further movement. An autonomous, unconscious feedback loop may thus develop which helps maintain immobility and disuse. Such a loop may sometimes play a major role in maintaining a vicious circle of pain and disuse. Although this can be considered psychosomatic, it is not simply a matter of belief and is not just in a person's head. Intervening in such a process requires having a different nervous system experience of the affected parts.

For example, my wife Susan once twisted her foot. She had pain and swelling and couldn't step onto it. After getting the foot and ankle x-rayed to rule out a fracture, she received the diagnosis of a moderate sprain. Nine days later, the swelling had subsided and she began to walk without crutches. However, she limped. I guided her through a process which involved performing a few small weight-shifting movements in different directions and then taking a few careful steps backwards. This took only a few minutes, after which she walked normally, no more limp, no pain.

Various sensory-movement techniques and hands-on methods (sometimes called "body work") exist. Whatever explanations they use (sometimes highly esoteric), practitioners of such methods succeed to a significant degree by establishing non-verbal trust and helping to reduce unnecessary guarding, increase movement and improve body awareness/sensation. Seeking out a skilled practitioner of one of these methods may help you begin to experience normal sensations and movements again.[3] See Chapter 12 for further discussion of body awareness and the role of reduced sensation following injury (especially the section, Sensory-Motor Amnesia).

Guarding and the Messages of Pain

Pain may have a useful message for you. Meditation teacher Milton Ward suggests that:

> Our instinctive being constantly emanates from and seeks a state of mental, emotional, physical and spiritual equilibrium. All pain is a request or demand to us (our minds) to help restore this equilibrium. It is a positive process.[4]

Guarding and the reduced sensation that accompanies it can thus involve a walling off of useful messages. You may need to bring your attention to your painful experience before you can move on:

> Instinct awareness, or pain awareness, can be remarkably helpful. One may experience the pain in both an immobile and an active state...If you have any long-term painful area, you may wish to try this right now. Hold your utmost concentration on the very core of the pain. Go deeper and deeper into the pain. Then, with ample patience respond to the intent of the pain...as precisely as you possibly can.[5]

Ward discusses how to use pain awareness during activities like walking:

> The key here is *not to wait*, as we normally do, for the pain to become severe before we allow it to rise to our consciousness. Instead we will watch for the very first scintilla of pain. And we will respond to this pain signal *no matter how slight it is*. The pain may ask you to slow down in your walking very considerably. It may demand that you release your abdomen. It may suggest a quite unexpected change in your leg or foot motion, or indicate that the physical problem is entirely related to a job situation or a per-

sonal anxiety. Or a thousand other possibilities...From a preventive standpoint, a great deal of misery could be avoided if we would pause briefly, whenever we are engaged in physical effort, to receive the instructions of our inner system.[6]

Index Your Symptoms

Developing the kind of pain awareness that Ward suggests involves the important relations among your attitudes, beliefs, expectations and your ongoing experience of pain (indicated in Figures 9.1 and 9.2). Talking about your symptoms in absolutistic, catastrophic and unrealistic ways will focus your attention and direct your ongoing efforts in ways that will likely prolong a vicious circle. Talking about your symptoms in non-absolutistic, non-catastrophic and realistic ways will help you to focus your attention and act in ways that promote mobility and recovery. Doing this depends upon guideline 3, learning how to index your pain and other symptoms, that is, to describe them as specifically as possible.

Indexing is a term from General Semantics, a practical philosophy concerned with promoting a scientific attitude in everyday life. In our introductory book on General Semantics, *Drive Yourself Sane*, my wife and I define indexing as "making our terms and statements as descriptive as possible by emphasizing individual differences as well as similarities."[7] This is important because:

> Our word categories lead us to focus on similarities rather than differences. Necessary and useful as this seems, however, no two individual people or things in any particular category are ever exactly the 'same'. No matter how similar they seem, differences remain.[8]

> The use of indexing comes from mathematics, where variables are given subscripts, for example x_1, x_2, x_3, etc. In our everyday language, the variables consist of the words

we use. We consider any statement at least somewhat indeterminate or 'meaningless' in an extensional ['fact'-based] sense until we specify our terms using indexes.

A client had been referred to Bruce with a diagnosis of "degenerative disc disease." Bruce explained to him that he needed to get a history and perform an examination. The client appeared impatient and asked, "Doesn't the referral tell you what to do?" Bruce explained that he viewed every person, even with the 'same' diagnosis, as an individual, different from anyone else. " 'Back'$_1$ is not 'back'$_2$," he said. Following this, the patient had no difficulty cooperating with the examination.[9]

Whatever the diagnosis, indexing reminds practitioners and their patients of each person's individuality. You are not a category or a statistic!

You can also index your symptoms according to where you experience them in your body. Pain$_{\text{in the middle of your back}}$ is not the same as pain$_{\text{along one side}}$ is not the same as pain$_{\text{in the buttock}}$ is not the same as pain$_{\text{into the thigh}}$, etc. Use the body diagram of Figure 10.1 to index your symptoms in this way.[10] Darken the area or areas where you experience pain. You can also indicate tingling ("pins and needles") with x's and numbness with o's. Changes in the location of your symptoms can provide important guidance when you are deciding to move in particular ways or to increase your activity.

In addition, you can use indexing to specify degrees of pain intensity and other symptoms. Some people talk and act as if pain is an either/or quality. "Either you have pain or you don't." This can lead to expecting complete and, sometimes, immediate relief. More realistically, you can index your pain as a process along a continuum. Pain scales like the ones in Figure 10.2 (used by many practitioners) allow you to rate your present pain from 0 (no pain) to 10 (the maximum you can imagine). Indexing pain in terms of a continuum of pain may

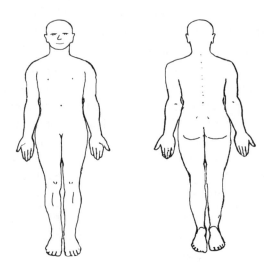

Figure 10.1 – Body Diagram

help you to have more reasonable expectations and to fully experience gradual changes. This may allow you to notice feeling better sooner as you work towards degrees of improvement rather than for all-or-nothing results.

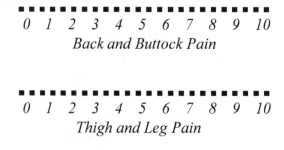

Figure 10.2 – Pain Scales

Another way to index your pain is to use chain indexes. Chain indexing involves indexing what you have already indexed or specified in order

> ...to indicate the effects of environmental conditions, location, etc. car_1 (with a full gas tank) will not work the same as car_1 (with an empty tank). We can note this as $car_{1,1}$ is not $car_{1,2}$.

> The chain index or, as General Semantics writer Kenneth Keyes called it, the "where" index, helps us to recognize "that any given person or thing may act differently when moved to a different place or placed in new circumstances."[11] Not only does back $patient_1$ not behave like back $patient_2$, but back $patient_1$ after walking for 30 minutes may have much less discomfort or no pain at all compared to back $patient_1$ after sitting slouched for 30 minutes. With chain indexing we can help ourselves and others to recognize the specific circumstances under which we feel pain, comfort, anxiety, enjoyment, etc. In this way we avoid acting as if every situation 'is' the same. [12]

Use the table on the next page to chain index ("where" index) your symptoms.[13] Make your comments as specific as possible as you describe what happens in each circumstance. For example, what type of chair are you sitting in when you feel better or worse? How long do you have to be sitting before you notice it worsening? In this way you will more easily be able to detect patterns that you can begin to make use of immediately to reduce your symptoms. You may also note any other activities that improve or worsen your symptoms.

The last form of indexing I will discuss is called *dating*. People, places and things change with time. Dating ("when" indexing [14]) gives you a way of indexing differences in time. As George Bernard Shaw noted, "The only man who behaves sensibly is my tailor; he takes my measure anew each time he sees me, whilst all the rest go on with their old measurements and expect them to fit me."[15] You can behave sensibly like

Activity	Better	Worse	Comments
Sitting			
Rising from sitting			
Standing			
Walking			
Bending			
First thing in a.m.			
As day progresses			
At end of day			
Lying			
Moving or at rest			

What Leaves You Better, Worse or In-Between? In What Way?

Shaw's tailor by attaching dates or "when" indexes to the terms and evaluations you use when describing your back pain. Consider the following questions which will help you take the time factor into account:

1. Is there any time during the day when I have no symptoms at all? In other words, are my symptoms intermittent or constant (felt all the time)?

2. How do my symptoms change according to the time of day or to what I'm doing?

3. How long have I had my symptoms?

4. In what location on my body did I first feel my symptoms?

5. Where are my symptoms located now?

6. Are my symptoms improving, worsening, or staying the same since they first started?

By indexing your pain and other symptoms in these various ways, you will become a better, more watchful observer of your pain. Instead of seeing pain as an 'enemy' to be avoided whenever possible, you will become more familiar with it in ways that can help you deal with it more successfully.

What Different Pains May 'Mean'

As a personal scientist, indexing your pain will help you to view your symptoms as controllable variables that can mean different things depending upon their changing location, intensity and presence in different situations at different times. If you have an activity-related (posture-movement) problem, you will be able to see some patterns in your symptoms related to your positions and movements, time of day, and other factors. Becoming a better observer of how your pain behaves in relation to different posture-movement factors will help you become more skillful in changing your actions in order to move towards recovery.

Here are some general rules that you can use to guide you:[16]

1.   You are moving towards recovery when your symptoms change in location in your body from peripheral to more central (closer to the spine).

2.   You are moving towards recovery if your symptoms are generally reducing in intensity. (Sometimes as symptoms reduce peripherally, they may increase centrally. In this case, the centralization probably indicates improvement even if the more central areas hurt more than they did before.)

3.   You are moving towards recovery when you can participate in more of your normal activities longer with fewer symptoms.

4.   You are moving towards recovery when your symptoms reduce in duration and frequency (from constant to intermittent and then, when intermittent, with shorter and less frequent periods.

5.   Intermittent pain felt only at the end range of a reduced range of motion indicates the existence of soft tissue adhesions and/or adaptive shortening. This kind of pain does not mean that damage is occurring. Rather, it may occur as a necessary part of improving range of motion after an injury has healed.

6.   Intermittent or constant pain which centralizes and reduces with a given activity and which is associated with an increase in mobility indicates the presence of a reducing joint displacement (McKenzie's derangement syndrome). The activity helps.

7.   Intermittent or constant pain which peripheralizes and increases with a given activity and which is associated with a reduction in mobility indicates the presence of an increasing joint displacement (McKenzie's derangement syndrome). The activity does not help.

8. Constant pain that does not improve with any activity or that worsens indicates the existence of a non-activity-related problem. It may indicate inflammation or some other condition that requires medical attention.

Explore Possibilities for Extending Your Spine

In this section, based on guideline 4, I describe a progression of positions and movements often used for treating relatively simple and common back problems. Although I cannot guarantee that it will work for you, if you first index your symptoms to establish a baseline and then ongoingly index the changes that occur while following the general rules above, you may be pleasantly surprised by the results that you achieve.

Overthrowing the Tyranny of Flexion

When I started out in the physical therapy profession, exercises for flexing the lower back (bending forwards) were a cornerstone of spinal rehabilitation. These often constituted what I call a "tyranny of flexion," because it was often assumed, with little questioning, that "If your back hurts, the first thing to try is bending forwards." The medical, chiropractic and physical therapy professions are now, in part, thanks to Cyriax, McKenzie and others, moving away from this emphasis.[17]

The tyranny of flexion encourages flexing the back even when it unintentionally may do harm. It is now more widely accepted that many people can rapidly improve by initially avoiding flexion and, instead, extending their backs. How then did flexion gain so much prominence as a treatment for back pain?

One major reason is that, for some people, there actually are times when flexing the back can be useful. A small number of people may actually improve by avoiding extension and doing flexion exercises.

There are also people like Paul, described in Chapter 3, who initially may be unable to extend and may need some time in the forward bent position in order to accommodate an apparent joint displacement which blocks the extension movement. Flexing the spine may provide temporary relief even though the problem may continue if they maintain the flexed position. Once they can extend the spine, they can often rapidly reduce their symptoms, especially if, for a while, they avoid letting their lower backs flex again. Once people in this situation have recovered sufficiently, they may benefit from flexing their spines in order to restore the full range of movement in their backs.

Other people have bone problems that result in a narrowing of the spaces for the spinal nerves (spinal stenosis). Some may have an actual fracture and slippage of the vertebrae, i.e., spinal bones (spondylolisthesis). People in this situation may benefit from not extending their backs and by flexing them to some degree in order to open the spaces for the nerves. (Of course, this depends on each person's individual response to the positions and movements.) In severe cases they may benefit from surgery.

Other people have gradually lost the ability to extend their spines. They have developed joint contractures and can't bend backwards without an uncomfortable stretch when they reach the limit of their restricted range of motion. They actually need to restore their lost range gradually. If they do not know how to do this correctly or if they get the wrong advice, they may interpret the pain or discomfort associated with the stretch as a sign not to continue. This type of problem has been encouraged by years of poor advice from prominent back pain experts.

Unfortunately, many doctors and therapists over-generalized from the successful uses of flexion, in order to bolster theories about posture and the inner workings of the back that now seem questionable.

In my personal library, I have a number of books by prominent back pain experts who have advocated controlled slumping (flexing the spine) as the recommended way for most people to sit comfortably. Some of these authorities have elaborated physiological and anatomical reasons why people should avoid extending their spines. According to them, one must do a pelvic tilt to slightly flex the spine before bending to lift.

One writer based this kind of advice on his observations of Indian peasants who squat with a slight flattening in their lower backs and were thought to have less back pain as a consequence. When an Indian physician was asked about this, he said, "Hell, those people are concerned about staying alive. They wouldn't complain about a little backache."[18]

If you observe people sitting, you will see that the longer they sit, the more likely they are to fall into a relaxed, slumped pattern. *They don't need advice from a book to do that!* People also will tend to move around in their chairs after a period of time spent sitting still. Some will actually arch their spines to stretch backwards. Could it be that they are getting some relief by extending their backs after a long period of slumping?

Despite years of poor advice, people have recovered from back pain. How many people would do better by getting individualized advice that takes into account the effects of positions and movements on their symptoms?

Extending Your Spine

I don't wish to establish a new tyranny of extension. I can't repeat too often (even if you feel tired of reading it) that treatment needs to be based on an individualized evaluation of the effects of positions and movements. Nonetheless, the extension routine that I will present here (derived from McKenzie's work) has often been found useful.[19]

There are some good theoretical reasons why extension can be helpful. As noted in the discussion of spinal anatomy in Chapter 5, the lumbar lordosis (hollow) constitutes a slightly extended position and serves a protective function for the spine. In addition, a modern way of life often leads to what McKenzie has called "the frequency of flexion." [20] The asymmetrical pressures of constant or frequent flexion can interfere with the mobility and nutrition of the discs. Extension movements can counterbalance these asymmetrical pressures and thus promote the normal nutrition, mobility and posture of the spine.

There also exist good empirical reasons for extending your spine. Extension often results in rapid relief of symptoms in people who appear to have soft tissue joint displacements involving the disc (McKenzie's derangement syndrome). Prior to McKenzie's work, this was observed by some often ignored practitioners who pioneered the use of spinal extension. As far back as 1962, Otto Reinert, D.C., wrote about his use of extension exercises for back pain. Another chiropractor, Fred Barge, questioned the use of flexion exercises and advocated spinal extension as well. [21] James Cyriax, M.D., also described the use of back extension exercise. [22] Combined with the postural advice contained in Part IV, you may find that extension works for you.

If you have sought medical advice as needed, ruled out red flag situations and developed a baseline by indexing your symptoms, you can proceed to explore the possibilities of extension for yourself by proceeding with the following positions and movements.

Of course, *I can't guarantee results*. There are too many variables and individual reactions involved. I cannot be there with you, the reader, to observe and guide what you do. This position and movement sequence will more likely work for you if :

  • You have pain in your back, buttocks and thighs either in the midline or equally on both sides, with no postural deformity.

  • You feel worse bending forwards.

  • You feel worse sitting, especially for long periods.

  • Standing in one place for long periods bothers you.

  • You get relief from your symptoms when you walk or lie down flat, especially on your stomach.

  • You feel better moving.

If so and if the pain that you feel is either constant or intermittent and goes no further than your buttock or thigh, with no other symptoms, start with exercise #1. You can do these exercises on a bed or the floor.

If you can't seem to get the results you want, seek further advice by seeing a health care practitioner experienced in this form of posture-movement therapy.

Exercise #1– Prone Lying

Exercise #1 (Figure 10.3) is simply the position of *lying prone* on your stomach. Remove eyeglasses if you wear them. You can rest your forehead or cheek on one or both hands or have your arms at your sides. Make yourself as comfortable as possible.

Notice where you feel your pain. Notice the furthest extent that you feel it from the middle of your back. After spending some time in this position, do you feel that lying prone makes the pain get worse in the most peripheral areas or spread out further towards your buttocks or legs? If so, you would do best to seek professional advice to get the added benefit of therapy as you get started.

If you feel no change after 5 minutes in this position or if you feel that the pain may be at least slightly better at the most peripheral areas of pain, go on to exercise #2, which is another static position, *prone on elbows*. You can move into it directly from the position you are in for exercise #1.

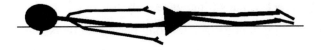

Figure 10.3 – Lying Prone

Exercise #2 – Prone on Elbows

Prop yourself up on your forearms so that your elbows are directly under your shoulders and your forearms and hands are resting on the surface in front of you. Keep your pelvis and legs on the floor and relax your back into a sagging position as much as you can. Remember to breathe. Remain in this position for two to five minutes (see Figure 10.4).

Again notice if you feel a reduction in the areas that were at the furthest extent of your symptoms. Perhaps the pains there have even disappeared and you feel symptoms closer to the midline of your spine. If so, great! You are ready to go on to exercise #3, also known as a prone press-up. If you feel no change in your symptoms you also can go on to #3.

If you feel worse in the same areas that hurt prior to doing this maneuver, you may need more time in the position of exercise #1. If you feel that your symptoms are peripheralizing, don't persist. Rather, lower yourself down to the prone position. You may find some useful advice on how to proceed in the section ahead labeled Problem-Solving Suggestions.

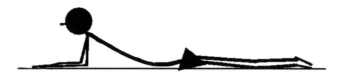

Figure 10.4 – Prone on Elbows

Exercise #3 – Prone Press-up

Return to the position in exercise #1. Place your open hands palm down under your shoulders or slightly to the front and side. This is the position in which you would put them if you were doing a standard push-up.

The difference with the press-up is that when you extend your arms straight, you allow your upper torso to lift while you leave your pelvis and legs on the floor. As you can see in the illustration (Figure 10.5), this will cause your lower back to sag into extension.

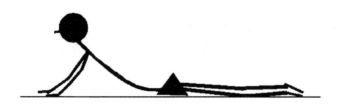

Figure 10.5 – Prone Press-up

Before you begin, take note of your symptoms. Notice the most peripheral location of the pain. Then perform one press-up. Go up as far as you can tolerate. To do the most good, you will need to get to your end range. Make sure that your arms do all the work. Let your buttocks relax and let your back sag. Remember to breathe.

You will need to repeat this movement about ten times, going as far as you can go each time. If with repetitions, you feel a lessening or disappearance of the most peripheral pain, even if you feel more pain at or closer to the center of your spine, this movement will probably help you to reduce and abolish your symptoms. Rest after doing ten.

When your arms have recovered, do another set of ten, monitoring your symptoms. The intensity and location of the pain are perceptions that you may be able to control through applying these movements. Your symptoms have centralized if the pain feels reduced and/or has disappeared peripherally while at the same time has either remained, increased or shifted more centrally (towards the middle of your spine).[23] If so then you can rest and repeat the exercise in sets of ten up to three or four times (depending on how much your arms can take). When you return to the prone resting position, you may be pleasantly surprised that you have no pain.

If so, what may have happened is that through your extension positions and movements you have squeezed the displaced fluid material of the disc towards the center of the joint. These fluid contents, which were distorting the joint and causing pain, have shifted into a more normal, neutral position in the joint.

However, even though you may have undone the displacement (derangement), the situation will not be stable at first. You will need to follow a systematic program of exercises and postural care for at least the next few days to turn this episode of pain into history.

Directional Preference

As McKenzie has noted, a joint displacement of the derangement syndrome type is characterized by the fact that symptoms can change location (centralize or peripheralize) fairly quickly. Moving in the direction that increases the derangement (usually flexion) creates a blockage to movement in the opposite direction (usually extension). Unfortunately, moving then in the direction of the blockage may also hurt.

Even though it may take some time, moving the spine in the initially blocked direction can lead to an overall reduction in pain and an increase in movement. If your pattern of symptoms is such that one direction of repeated movements increases and one direction decreases your symptoms and ability to move, you demonstrate, what McKenzie calls, a *directional preference* in your movement pattern.[24] This characterizes a derangement syndrome.

While it will lead to long-term comfort, finding the directional preference may take some skill since it often will initially be blocked and painful to move in that direction. If you have responded positively to exercises #1, #2 and #3, you have a directional preference for spinal extension. If this doesn't seem clear, see the next section for suggestions.

If you go away from the directional preference and flex your spine too soon, the unstable material in the disc may have a chance to displace again. Until things have settled and the formerly displaced tissues heal sufficiently, you will need to *maintain your lordosis curve at all times!* In the following chapters on posture and body mechanics, I will provide some concrete suggestions on how to do this. Consult especially the sections on sitting and folding in Chapter 13.

Problem Solving Suggestions

It seems appropriate here to provide some guidance for those of you who do not get adequate relief of symptoms with the prone progression. I will add a few tips here that you can attempt on your own. If these don't seem to work, you will benefit from getting professional advice.

Some people with derangement type symptoms may find that they cannot lie prone without increasing or peripheralizing their back pain. Similarly, when standing you may find it difficult to straighten up or you may feel blocked in bending backwards.

In this case, you can start by lying prone with one or two pillows under your abdomen. Find out how many you need in order not to increase your symptoms. You may need to reduce the pillows very gradually (it may take a half hour or more) until you can do exercise #1 and lie flat with no increase or peripheralization of pain.

Sometimes the deranged fluid material of the disc may just need time to redistribute to a new position. For this very reason, you may also need to give more time to each exercise before moving on to the next one. If you move too quickly in the blocked direction, you may simply be squeezing the deranged area of the joint without reducing the derangement. If you follow this suggestion and still do not get relief, please seek further advice from an appropriately trained practitioner.

It is also possible that you feel your symptoms more towards one side, where the derangement has occurred. Movement in the extension direction may squeeze without reducing the distorted tissues of the disc, while flexion will unsqueeze but tend to increase the extent of the derangement.

If so and if you have an obvious deformity and find yourself bent or twisted to one side as a result of this back pain episode, you had best get personal help from a spinal care practitioner. If you have no obvious deformity, however, you may want to try the following, if you can do exercise #1 with no increase in symptoms, even though the other exercises in the prone progression have not helped.

With this type of problem you will probably have a directional preference towards the painful side. To determine if this is so, lie prone (on your stomach) and shift your hips towards the painfree side. This will shift your trunk and lower back towards the painful side. If the painful side is to the right, shifting the hips to the left makes the trunk shift toward the painful right side. If you have pain on the left you will need to shift in the opposite direction.

You will know this maneuver is working if you feel that the pain centralizes. You can then perform the prone progression with your body shifted in this way. If you find that this doesn't work seek professional advice.[25]

A few people who do not respond well to extension will have back pain with blocked forward bending and a full or increased lordosis. Those with this kind of condition will not improve by doing exercises that encourage extension. Their directional preference is for flexion. Exercise #5, Flexion in Lying, likely will reduce and abolish symptoms in this case. Postural advice will need to be modified from what is given for posterior derangements. Again it will be best to get this evaluated professionally.

It is also possible that you are not responding because you do not have a mechanical back problem. Alternatively, you may have one of the less common types of mechanical problems noted in the last chapter. An activity-related (mechanical) evaluation and trial period of treatment can help you to find solutions for your problem.

Exercise #4 - Extension in Standing

Assuming that you have been successful with the previous steps of exercises #1, #2 and #3 (the prone progression), get yourself up slowly and carefully from the floor or bed. Make sure that you maintain your lordosis while you bring yourself up to standing. Walk around a bit to find out how you feel. You may feel painfree or at least much improved. As I mentioned, you will need to be extremely vigilant about your posture and movements for at least the next day or two, avoiding any hint of flexion in your lumbar spine.

Going through the prone progression and doing the press-ups as often as possible (every two to three hours) will help you to get to a painfree state and to maintain the painfree state until the tissues stabilize. It will also help you to return to a painfree state if your back begins to hurt again.

If you are in a situation where you cannot lie down to do the press-ups, then exercise #4, extension in standing, can be done as a substitute. In addition, if you have been sitting (even if you sit correctly with a lordosis), get up frequently before you begin to feel any return of symptoms, or when you feel just a hint of their return, and do five or six repetitions of exercise #4 as a preventive measure.

To do exercise #4, spread your feet shoulder width apart. Make fists and place them in your lumbar area approximately at waist level. Your fists will serve as leverage points for the movement. Notice if you have any symptoms and, if so, where they are located.

Now bend backwards, extending your lumbar area, while continuing to look forwards with your eyes open (this is a lower back, not a neck, exercise). Make sure your knees remain easy and unlocked and go slowly enough so that you can maintain your balance. Extend as far as you can, noting any changes in your symptoms. Repeat ten times. When you stop, you should not feel any worse than you did before you began.

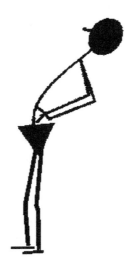

Figure 10.5—Extension in Standing

If you were able to get positive results with the prone progression but find that you feel worse after doing this exercise, you will need to work for awhile lying prone. For some reason, you may be particularly sensitive to the effect of your upper body weight in the standing position.

If you feel that extension is limited and you notice end range pain that doesn't get worse with repetitions, you have stiffness in the direction of extending your back.

I have seen this condition quite often and attribute it to "the tyranny of flexion," having been told for years that flexion is 'good' and lordosis and extension are 'bad'. If you have lost the ability to extend your back, you will need to work on both prone and standing extension to recover your lost mobility. A thorough evaluation of the effects of positions and movements on your symptoms may help you to deal with this condition.

Recovering Function

Once constant pain has become intermittent and intermittent pain has become minimal, it may be time to begin the process of recovering function. If your derangement has gotten reduced, the displaced material will have returned to its normal position. By continuing with the appropriate movements and correct posture, you may have maintained the reduction for at least a few days. In this case, you no longer need to do the extension exercises every couple of hours.

As noted in the previous chapter, after an injury the process of healing continues in its later phases through the formation of scar tissue. The scar provides a connective tissue repair of the damaged and torn tissues. However, if inadequate stress is placed on the scar while it is forming and maturing the repair will be stiff and weak. In other words, an adhesion will have formed. Your muscles may also have gotten adaptively shortened

So if you have been following the instructions above and avoiding flexion, you will need to begin moving in this direction again. How do you know whether it's time? You can tell by performing a repeated movement test of flexion in lying. This is exercise #5.

Exercise #5 - Flexion in Lying

First do one set of press-ups as usual. You should have no pain with this, except perhaps some end range stiffness if you are one of those who has lost some extension mobility.

Following this, turn over and lie down on your back. Notice if you have any symptoms. You should still feel painfree. Then bend your knees one at a time and one at a time lift your feet from the surface you are lying on. Each knee should come up high enough so that you can grab hold of each one firmly. From this starting position use your hands to assist and guide you as you pull both knees at the same time towards your chest as far as they'll go. Your tail bone and lower back will lift from the surface. Then return to the starting position.

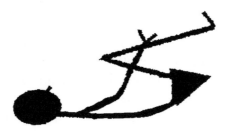

Figure 10.6 — Flexion in Lying

If you feel some discomfort, at what point in the exercise do you feel it? Note if you feel pain during the movement (somewhere in mid-range) or at the end range of the movement. Repeat the movement about ten times, making sure that you go to the maximum of the end range that you can. If you feel pain during the movement that seems to be worsening, stop and proceed to do more extensions. You are not ready.

However, if you have pain related to stiffened adhesions or adaptively shortened muscles, you will feel no pain during movement. Instead you will feel some pulling pain or discomfort at end range that will stop when you get out of that position. You will also feel no worse, which in this case means painfree, after ten repetitions.

Now turn over once again to lie prone and do another set of press-ups. You should still be able to do these as before to full range with no pain. If so, you have a "green light" to proceed with the process.[26]

If you feel anything different and notice pain during press-ups that remains after stopping, go through another prone progression. You may need to stay there awhile and do several sets of press-ups.

This is a "red light" situation for recovering function with flexion exercises. Since you were able to do extension in lying before with full movement and no pain, the flexion movement has likely caused the blocked and painful extension. In other words, you still have a directional preference for extension. Reduction of the derangement is not yet fully stable. Continue with the extension program as before.

You may find that things don't seem this clear. For example, you may find that the flexion exercise feels uncomfortable during movement as well as end range, but that your ability to do the extensions afterwards is unimpaired. You can treat this as a "yellow" light, and cautiously proceed with the instructions for recovering function with flexion exercises.

If you are able to proceed with flexion exercises, you can begin recovering function by starting with two or three periods of flexion exercises (ten repetitions) per day. Initially, do a set of press-ups first. *Always* follow the flexion exercise with a set of press-ups. You also should wait for several hours after getting up before doing any flexion. Since you have increased pressures inside the discs on first getting up, flexing too soon in the day has a potential for causing a new displacement.

You should continue with extension in lying and standing as needed, and with proper body mechanics. You can begin to return to the normal activities that you may have stopped or reduced when your back was hurting.

Continuing Your Progress

Flexion exercises can prove useful if flexion is stiff and limited and thus interferes with your everyday activities. Flexion in lying can be done safely by following the guidelines noted above. There are more advanced types of flexion exercises that may help you further recover function if needed. However, I do not include them here. As Cyriax noted, because of the "tyranny of flexion" many people mistakenly believe that "no-one is 'fit' unless he can bend and touch his toes."[27] Nonsense! There is no particular need for you to bend down and touch your toes if you have no other problems.

In many cases, I believe that the flexion in lying exercise will suffice to help recover function. If you feel that you need to go further with flexion exercises, first get a proper evaluation with repeated movement testing that can help you assess your actual need to increase that movement and the safety in doing so.

Flexion exercises need to be done with caution, using the traffic light approach mentioned previously. As a general guideline, if you have had an episode of back pain which has benefited from extension exercises, you will be well served by including a healthy dose of extension after doing these other movements.

The position and movement sequence using extension was devised by McKenzie for the simplest and most common types of lower back pain. If my descriptions seem to fit your type of problem, you may be able to reduce and abolish your symptoms by working in the way suggested here.

For more detailed advice however, you will best be served by consulting with a practitioner who can evaluate your condition and determine specifically what you need for an individualized, self-care exercise program.

Either from reading this book or getting the advice of a qualified spinal care practitioner, you can learn how to help yourself feel better now. By learning self-care procedures, you will have a skill that you can use in the future. What worked for you this time is quite likely to work for you again in the event of a future episode. Whenever you feel the onset of pain, you can act immediately to cut it short and reduce the intensity and duration of symptoms. If you have had a history of recurring back pain episodes, it may be possible to reduce the frequency of recurrences. You can research this for yourself!

Improve Your Posture-Movement Habits

Guideline #5 for dealing with back pain suggests that you "Improve your posture-movement habits." Although dealing with your posture may not be sufficient in itself for treating back pain, it remains a necessary adjunct to any comprehensive therapy. Whatever the activity-related problem, your posture-movement habits will surely have a major effect on your level of pain and well-being. Poor posture will further aggravate any other soft tissue problems that exist. Good posture will reduce stress. In the next section of the book, I discuss some basic principles of better body use to apply when you experience and are recovering from back pain. They also may help reduce the probability of future problems.

Part IV

Education Solutions

Prevent the things you have been doing
and you are half way home.
- F. M. Alexander[1]

Chapter 11

Essentials of Body Mechanics

The Power of Posture

Chiropractors, orthopedic surgeons and physical therapists generally agree (imagine that!) that posture constitutes an important factor in overcoming back pain.[1] By now, you may at least have an inkling of the importance of body mechanics and use in dealing with your back problem.

You posture-movement habits may produce or reduce pain due to stress and strain on normal tissues. Your posture-movement habits can also aggravate or reduce the pain due to pre-existing soft-tissue problems.

Changing these habits ultimately does not depend upon treatment or therapy. Ultimately it depends upon education and steadfast intent. In this chapter, I provide you with some essentials of body mechanics. I will also discuss some of the constraints and requirements for learning better posture-movement habits. These will help you understand and use four educational guidelines for using yourself better. These education guidelines are listed at the end of the chapter and discussed in individual chapters to follow.

Essentials of Body Mechanics

Good posture-movement habits ("body mechanics" or "use") involve coordinating the parts and the whole of yourself in such a way that there is minimal possibility of damage to the muscles, joints, etc., and maximal performance efficiency.

Joel E. Goldthwait, M.D., an orthopedic surgeon, provided an analysis of what good use entails in his seminal textbook, *Essentials of Body Mechanics*. The following discussion is indebted to Goldthwait's work.

As Goldthwait and his co-authors noted, every one of the joints of your body has a range of motion, the total amount of mobility in any direction. This range can vary among individuals depending on the shapes of the joint surfaces, the elasticity of ligaments and the stabilizing ability of the muscles.

Extend and then flex your wrist. Notice the complete range of motion possible in either direction. As noted in Chapter 9, the so-called normal range of motion of any joint or set of joints, such as the wrist or spine, can get reduced for a variety of reasons.

Whatever your particular range of motion happens to be, when you get to the end range or furthest point of the motion only a slight amount of extra movement or "play" in the joint is possible. You can observe this joint play by applying a little external pressure at the end range of either movement of the wrist.

This kind of end range pressure done in a controlled manner, may be necessary and useful to reveal and to treat soft tissue contractures. However, keeping a joint at the extreme of end range may cause undesirable pain.

Initially, such pain may simply provide a warning signal. When you bent your finger backwards until you felt discomfort, you experienced such a warning pain at the extreme end range of your finger joints.

If applied too strongly, too long or too often during your everyday activities, such end range forces may increase the likelihood of injury.

On the other hand, when you allow your joints to work more of the time in more neutral positions and not at the extremes of end range, you allow what Goldthwait called a "factor-of-safety motion." Think of a joint as a hinge. If a door is opened as far as its hinge allows, a surprisingly small application of force might easily damage the hinge or break it. The same force applied to the halfway open door would have little effect.

If a joint is not locked at end range, it has some leeway to move without creating strain. This factor-of-safety also allows your muscles to have more of an ability to exert a protective, stabilizing influence on the affected joints. As Goldthwait put it, "Good body mechanics imply that all the joints of the body are used in such a position in relation to their total range of motion that the possibility of further motion in either direction—the factor-of-safety motion—is always present." [2]

The factor-of-safety is not just about the range of motion within a single joint. As I mentioned previously, any movement involves a chain of connections throughout the musculoskeletal system. Any single joint thus can gain a factor-of-safety from a conscious, flexible linkage with other joints. This linkage provides a factor of efficiency as well.

Notice the difference between examples *A* and *B* on the next page. *A* illustrates a person inattentively bending forwards and flexing his spine in order to pick up a package from the floor. *B* illustrates someone picking up a package by thoughtfully allowing the spine and torso to lengthen while folding the hips, knees and ankles over the base of support of the feet.

A shows a method of movement that 'isolates' the back from the rest of the body. The joints of the spine appear close to a flexed end range position. The hips and knees are also locked close to end range positions. These positions allow for little factor-of-safety motion for the spine. As a result, the lower back carries an excessive amount of the forces of lifting. You know what can happen then!

With *B*, the forces of lifting are distributed more evenly throughout the musculoskeletal system. Supporting muscles stabilize the joints of the spine within more neutral positions and away from end range. A greater factor-of-safety and efficiency exists. The back, hips, knees, ankles, the strong muscles of the lower extremities, etc., work together to share the effort. This allows the load to be lifted more safely and easily. The back 'gets by with a little help from its friends'.

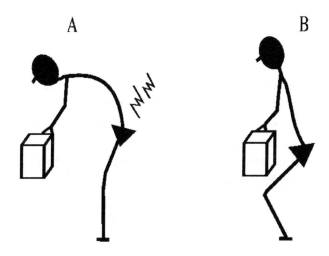

Figure 11.1 — Poor Vs. Good Body Mechanics

When you allow the normal curves in your spine to be present without reducing or exaggerating them, you allow more of this factor-of-safety and efficiency to be present. In order to do this you need to engage your other joints more when squatting, lifting, etc. In this way, your spine and torso will work at their optimal length and stability. You will function closer to your full stature with the least amount of effort necessary.

Posture, Movement and Modern Life

Such optimal movement may exist in a healthy young child. Constantly active, she will tend to move as her focus of interest changes. Given a short attention span, this likely means that she moves a lot! The *postural variety* resulting from this more or less constant movement means that she does not spend a great deal of time in one position, hanging at the end range of her joints. Even though her posture is not conscious, it may appear quite good.

When she begins going to school, working with computers, watching more television, etc., this situation can change. Spending more time sitting in chairs in static positions will lead to *postural monotony*. She will probably spend more time with her joints at or near end range, with a reduced factor-of-safety motion in her joints. The child's posture-movement habits, again not conscious, will begin to look more like that of the sedentary adults around her.

The kind of sedentary adult life-style that a child can 'slump' into is based to a large extent on the conditions of modern life. Too many people sit too much of the time. We live in a car-culture where walking is usually not a required, or sometimes even a safe, way to get from home to work to stores, chores, friends, play, etc. More and more people spend hours a day sitting in front of computer screens at work and play.

Even those who have jobs that involve more movement and activity, i.e., gardeners, waitresses, factory workers, etc., often end up doing repeated activities involving stereotyped movements and slumped positions that reduce postural variety and the factor-of-safety in their joints.

As we have already noted, variations of movement and pressure are required to maintain adequate circulation to the discs. Postural monotony in asymmetrical, usually flexed positions thus interferes with the optimal nutrition of the spine.

The 'cure' for an inactive life-style often involves recreational exercise such as running, aerobics, weight training, etc. Yet working out at the health club can have its own perils. Posture-movement habits developed during the course of everyday life do not suddenly get dropped when someone exercises. Just take a look in any fitness center at the people sitting crouched over their exercise bikes. Unfortunately, exercises that get taken up to improve fitness may actually imperil one's musculoskeletal health because they are done with insufficient attention to body mechanics and use.

Body Mechanics and Exercise

The basics of optimal body use (we might call it the "ethics of the body") have relevance across different times and cultures. Although no two people are exactly the same in all respects, we humans do share a common structure and deal with gravity and other forces in a similar way.

However, schools of thought differ as to how to achieve this optimal body use. Traditional rehabilitation practice has focused on correcting posture and body mechanics through stretching and strengthening exercises. This remains a major emphasis of many health-care practitioners. Though such exercises may help, emphasizing exercise to improve body mechanics seems fundamentally mistaken.[3]

Of course, you do need a minimal level of strength and range of motion to maintain optimal posture. However, it is not clear the extent to which exercises to strengthen the relevant muscle groups and improve joint range of motion are necessary to achieve and maintain this condition.[4] Even if you exercise with the most advanced machines to superbly stretch and strengthen your back, butt, abdominal muscles, etc., this won't suffice to keep you from slumping when you're sitting in a restaurant eating your soup.

Every sports trainer knows about the "specificity of training." Working out and stretching may be important prerequisites for skilled performance. Eventually though, an athlete needs to practice the actual activities of his particular sport in order to train the musculoskeletal system to its peak. To get good at a skill, you need to practice that skill in the way you'll actually want to perform it.

In a similar way, to get good at the skill of using yourself with better body mechanics when you sit, stand, squat, etc., you need to practice this skill when you are sitting, standing, squatting, etc.

Sometimes a person's posture does seem to improve to some degree after starting a course of exercises. Part of this may come about as an indirect side effect of increasing general activity and thus reducing postural monotony, improving energy level and conditioning important muscles.

Postural improvement, to the extent that it occurs in this case, may also come about because the person has somehow developed greater body awareness in the course of exercise training. Good fitness trainers will consistently emphasize the importance of proper technique and form while exercising.[5]

The importance of learning good use has begun to get a glimmer of recognition with an approach to back rehabilitation called "spinal stabilization," which retrains a person to control and maintain a stable position of the spine while performing various exercises.[6]

Experience and research with the Alexander Technique indicate that focusing on exercising the specific muscles involved is not necessary to establish this control. This is consistent with Perceptual Control Theory as well. Learning how to support yourself in an upright position in sitting primarily depends on your desire to sit better, on developing a clear and accurate internal standard of upright posture and on actually spending time working to perceive yourself sitting in this way.

It's a 'spiral' process of circular causation that gets refined and developed with time and practice. Supporting yourself in a lengthened and upright manner, you will automatically exercise and condition the muscles that you need to support yourself in that position. This, in turn, will make it easier for you to support yourself in a more lengthened and upright manner.

'Exercise' systems such as Hatha Yoga, Qigong and Tai Chi also go beyond a purely muscle training approach. Questionable metaphysics aside, these disciplines have much to offer because they can provide a number of interesting ways to develop the kind of awareness and control of body use that I've been talking about here.[7]

It may seem that I am 'down' on exercise. This is not the case. In no way do I wish to discourage you from working out in a gym, if that's what you want to do. Weight training, aerobics (cardio-pulmonary) exercises of various kinds, and stretching can benefit you greatly. They can benefit you even more, while further reducing the probability of injuring yourself when doing them, if you apply an awareness of body mechanics as you exercise and in your daily living.

Learning Better Use

Many spinal care practitioners consider it important to help their clients with their body mechanics and use. It has been shown that simple instructions in posture and body use can make at least an incremental difference in how one feels and moves. This is especially so with people in pain who feel especially motivated to sit and move 'correctly'.[8]

However, facilitating deeper change in a person's manner of use requires something more than an instruction booklet or the cursory instruction usually available in a busy physical therapy, chiropractic or medical clinic.

An important constraint to learning involves your 'feeling' of what is 'right' or 'natural'. Your habits of use developed mostly unconsciously over the course of your life. In terms of the perceptual control model discussed in Chapter 7, you likely have your postural 'thermostat' set at a particular level that is mostly a function of what you've gotten used to. Like Jeremy, the young man in Chapter 4 whom I attempted to help with his posture, what feels right to you may not actually be very good for you. Your bad habits may feel 'right' simply because you're used to them.

Related to this, you quite likely also have gaps of awareness as well as misconceptions and faulty perceptions in relation to your body. Our perceptions and ideas function like internal cognitive maps of our bodies and environments.[9] It may be something of a shock to you to realize that your perceptual map of your body is not the same as your body itself. Like any map, it necessarily leaves out some things and may in fact be highly inaccurate. This is just what F.M. Alexander found when working on himself.

For example, when students are guided manually to unlock their knees and hips and stand with greater length and balance, they often report at first that they feel as if they are leaning far forwards. A glance in the mirror demonstrates to them that this is not so. Becoming aware of this 'mismatch' between what you see and what you kinesthetically sense can serve a very useful purpose. Realizing the fallibility of your senses can remind you to continue to check, refine and improve your use. In this way your body sense can become more reliable with time.

These constraints limit what can be learned from a book. Even with the most detailed written instructions possible, I have no knowledge of how any one reader may translate these instructions and apply them. Intensive, one-on-one instruction is required for learning consistent, long-term and habitual better use. Nothing can match personal instruction from someone knowledgeable. Here we enter the realm of the Alexander Technique of posture-movement education.

In my own practice, clients with back pain get some of the Alexander Technique educational work to supplement the activity-related therapy I provide. In addition, anyone who is interested can take PostureSense® group classes (based on the Alexander Technique) to learn and practice essential body mechanics.[10] Those who wish to go still further can take individualized lessons in the Alexander Technique of posture-movement education. Alexander Technique training in mindful body mechanics provides one of the best ways I know to learn long term habits of better body use.[11]

Research by Wilfred Barlow, M.D., David Garlick, M.D., Frank Pierce Jones, Ph.D., Chris Stevens and others has demonstrated some of the effects of Alexander Technique lessons. These writers have also discussed the requirements for learning better use in everyday life.

Learning better body use involves actually experiencing better use. With exposure and repetition, perceiving good use in your own body will lead to your developing a reliable internal reference standard for good use.[12] This may seem like a bit of a "Catch 22." To learn good use, you need to experience good use. To experience good use, you need to learn good use. Personal instruction can help you resolve this apparent dilemma.

The teacher must provide a good enough personal standard in his or her own posture-movement behavior to adequately provide this instruction. The teacher's body use sets a visible example of poise for the student. The teacher's good body mechanics are also conveyed non-verbally through manual contact with the student. This skill requires a level of non-verbal art that involves a significant amount of training to acquire.

There also are internal requirements on the part of the student of good use. Developing better postural control depends on your will to learn it. You need to want to develop better use. This desire will keep you on track towards your ultimate goal of feeling and moving better.

As you begin to observe yourself more, you may discover a certain resistance in yourself to doing so. Except for exceptional times, paying attention to your use may not seem 'natural'. On the other hand, some of you reading this may already be paying too much attention to yourselves in ways that are not helpful.

If you find that you are getting obsessive about your posture, it may be useful to forget about it for awhile. Spastic self-preoccupation is not advisable. Avoid tying up your brain in a pretzel by trying to sit up 'straight'.[13]

It may help if you realize that your habits of use are related to your habits of attention. I want to help you learn *constructive* conscious control of yourself. This means that with the proper instruction and practice, you will be able to expand your field of attention to include your 'outward' focus on whatever end you want to achieve (what you are doing) along with an 'inward' awareness of how you are doing what you are doing (your use). This 'ought' to and can be a relaxed, even interesting, way of doing things.

How much are you allowing the optimal length of your spine, right where you are now? If you ask yourself this question with an inquiring attitude, what kind of difference can it make in your reading position now? This kind of awareness can become easier with practice.

This awareness involves being able to apply your improved posture-movement patterns to your activities on a moment-to-moment basis. Doing this requires a set of cognitive skills called "thinking in activity" by the philosopher John Dewey, who was a student of the Alexander Technique. These skills of awareness include the ability to "inhibit" and "direct," discussed in Chapter 4 and further explained in the next chapter.

To best assure that you understand the basic principles of body use, I recommend individualized lessons in the Alexander Technique with a qualified teacher. These lessons can assist you to more deeply internalize a new body awareness and moment-to-moment better use. This can set you off in the right direction for continuing on your path of self-care.

As I said before, improving your body mechanics is not an all or nothing process. I have observed that the four-session PostureSense® class and/or a short course of ten or fewer

Alexander Technique lessons can lead to significant observable changes in a motivated student's habits. There are also other therapeutic systems and exercise approaches that may help you to improve your use.

Even given the superiority of personal instruction, working on yourself with written instructions from a book may also help you to some degree. In the next several chapters, I will present four general rules of 'mindful' body mechanics and some ways to apply them in your daily activities. These rules have been developed as flexible guidelines for you to apply as you work on your own to improve your use.

Here are the guidelines:

1. *Make body awareness a daily practice.* (Chapter 12)

2. *Experience your full stature every day as often as you can.* (Chapter 13)

3. *Design your personal environment for better use.* (Chapter 14)

4. *Practice postural variety in your daily life.* (Chapter 15)

How can you apply these to begin to move yourself towards better body use in your daily life?

Chapter 12

Practice Body Awareness

The first guideline for better body use is: *Make body awareness a daily practice.*

The Limits of Awareness

Practicing body awareness may not seem easy at times. We all have a certain amount of psychological inertia. We tend to move in the well-worn grooves of what we give our habitual attention to and what we ignore. We often function in a limited state of awareness that psychologist Ellen Langer calls "mindlessness."[1]

In such a state, our attention runs more or less on automatic and our behavior seems less-than-optimally sensitive to the conditions surrounding us and inside of us. At such times, our experience may seem like something that happens to us, not something that we have an opportunity to shape as we like.

On the other hand, we also can function at times with a less automatic, more alert state of awareness in which we are more open to what is going on around and in us, i.e., Langer's "mindfulness." We can look at things from more than one perspective.

At such times, novelty and the present context become important. We are open to new information. What we attend to becomes more something we do and less something that happens to us.

The difference between this alert state of awareness and the more automatic state of attention noted above may be a matter of need, interest or skill, among other factors.

Someone who likes melons and knows a lot about produce may go to a food store with melon on his list, look at the different melons, sniff and poke one and then another until he finds one that seems just right. Someone else, with less interest and knowledge and more distractions may go to get a melon and put the first one he comes to into his basket. When asked why he picked that one he may say, "A melon is a melon."

I have been describing relative states perhaps on opposite ends of a continuum of consciousness. Indeed, a certain amount of automatism seems like a necessary feature of our cognitive landscape.

As a mapping system, the brain cannot include in our awareness all of the information that it processes. Our awareness, as Korzybski pointed out, is necessarily an abstracting process—as the brain/nervous system selects some experiences to attend to, it filters out other aspects.[2] We often use repetitive patterns. We can thus save time and energy by putting our information abstracting equipment on automatic.

In this way our habits free us from having to focus our limited attention on repetitive tasks and concerns. However, we need the ability to go beyond our habits, to extend the limits of our awareness. Otherwise we can lose our ability to respond effectively to new and different situations that arise. Instead of serving us, our habits can become our masters.

Experience and Words

In order to improve your posture-movement habits, you need to become more mindful of what you do and how you do it (your tensions, body posture, etc.). This will require that you bring yourself out of the automatic mode of awareness more often.

One important distinction to remember when doing this is the difference between the world of non-verbal experience and the world of words.[3]

Try this experiment: Pinch your ear lobe! Do it now. Now keep pinching it and say, "I'm pinching my earlobe." Now stop pinching your ear lobe and say "I'm pinching my ear lobe." (You will not get any benefit from this if you don't actually do it. Words will not suffice.)

This experiment illustrates that the territory of the non-verbal experience of the pinch is not the same as the word-maps you may use to talk about it. Whatever you say about your experience, for example "ouch" or "it hurts," is *not* it.

Nonetheless, in various ways, your habitual beliefs, embodied in your way of talking about your experience, can direct what you do and thereby experience ongoingly. This happens through the circular, feedback process of perceptual control discussed previously. How you talk about things will set the internal standards or reference levels that will determine what perceptions you control for. In this way, your habitual mode of awareness can be perpetuated by what you say to yourself.

Simply having an awareness of this can make a difference in what and how you experience. You can discover more accurate, more useful ways of talking to yourself about yourself and what you experience, including your experience of pain.

For example, I once taught at a seminar held on a college campus. My wife and I were staying in a room in the college dormitory, near the designated women's bathroom. The men's room was a long way down the hallway in the opposite wing of the dormitory. I woke up in the middle of the night with a full bladder. Trudging out to the hall, I looked around and briefly contemplated using the women's room but decided to "do the right thing" and began the long trek to the men's room. The trip started out with a sense of urgency that wasn't helped by my telling myself, "Oh boy, this is awful. I don't know if I can hold it… ohh, it's uncomfortable…it's such a long way down the hall." However, having gotten in the habit of listening to myself and knowing that what I said to myself could make a difference in what I experienced, I began a different kind of self-talk. "My muscles work very well to hold things. What wonderful control. I can make it to the bathroom. I'd prefer not having to walk so far, but it's not so bad." Let me tell you, I felt very proud of my self-talk that night.

As general semanticist and psychologist Wendell Johnson noted years ago, your most enchanted listener remains yourself. What you say to yourself can sometimes affect what you experience. Johnson illustrated the point with this light verse:

> A rose with onion for its name
> Might never, never smell the same —
> And canny is the nose that knows
> An onion that is called a rose.[4]

Sensory Awareness

Even though we live and experience our lives on what Korzybski called "the silent, unspeakable" non-verbal level of existence, it seems that we are endlessly talking to ourselves. As suggested in the last section, our self-talk can keep us stuck in habitual, unconscious, unhelpful patterns if it is based mostly on unquestioned verbal definitions. On the other hand, if we talk to ourselves in factual ways that keep us open to the possibilities of new experience, we can adapt better to what is happening within and around us.

Eventually, a large part of living in this fact-based, experiential way (what general semanticists call an "extensional orientation") involves not just learning how to talk differently to ourselves but also how to turn down the volume of the words inside our heads. This means practice at looking, listening, tasting, feeling, etc., at the silent, unspeakable level. Turning down the volume of our internal chatter gives us more of a chance to receive new signals and thus to learn new things about the world and ourselves. Not only can this make us more adaptable to changing circumstances; it can also make life more fun.

An approach to living that offers some suggestions for doing this is the educational practice known as "Sensory Awareness" taught by Charlotte Selver. Selver, who now has a number of her students teaching this work, studied with Elsa Gindler, a physical education teacher in Germany in the early part of the twentieth century.[5]

Gindler had no effective medical treatment available when she contracted tuberculosis. She had little money and could not afford going to a sanatorium, which at the time, before the advent of effective antibiotic treatment, was where such patients went in order to improve their chances of survival. She did, however, have some hope that by observing herself, how she breathed and moved, she might at least not interfere with whatever capacity her system had to fight the infection.

She found that when she could get out of her own way, remain present here and now, and keep her attention on the actual processes of breathing and moving, she could function more easily.

Some time later, when she encountered her doctor in the street, he seemed surprised at her appearance of good health. Indeed Gindler lived for many more years and taught others, including Selver, her unique form of psycho-physical education.

Sensory Awareness work (which I studied with Charlotte Schuchardt Read, a student of Selver) uses questions and experiments to direct your attention non-verbally to what is going on in and around you. In this way, you can learn to stay more in the present as you sense your organism-as-a-whole-in-an-environment connections.

I would like to give you a taste of a sensory awareness experiment right now. As you read the following, allow yourself time to observe and respond:

What are you doing right now, non-verbally?

How can you allow yourself to feel the support of what holds you up?

How much do you need to hold yourself up?

Where do you feel unnecessary tensions?

Do you feel tension in your jaw?

Do you feel tension in your face?

Where do you feel ease?

How clearly can you feel yourself breathing?

Remember that directing your attention in this way takes time. When you focus unnecessarily on labeling and explaining, you may miss something important going on in and around you.

Listen to whatever sounds come to you right now...Do you find yourself labeling what you hear? Listen again and this time, if you begin to label sounds, just notice that you are doing it and come back to the sounds again...

Touch the cloth of your clothes. Notice the sensations in your fingers, your hands. Allow the sensations to travel where they will. Move to a different part of your clothes. Notice any different sensations.

Choose something to look at. Without words, take in what comes to your eyes. Continue looking; what else comes to you?

Get up and walk around. Sense the movement of your feet and legs, the movement of your arms, the shifts of your torso.

Consider the sounds, sights, and aromas around you as structures to explore. Pick an object, such as a stone or a pencil. Examine it closely, silently for several minutes. Use 'all' of your senses: see, hear, touch, taste, move, etc. How well can you do this without labeling or describing?

You may find that you quickly fall into speech, perhaps talking to yourself about something else. Perhaps you scold yourself for not performing the task 'correctly'. You may also find yourself congratulating yourself verbally for remaining on the non-verbal level. If you find yourself doing these things, just notice it and go on. With practice, you'll find it easier to stay focused on the non-verbal level.

You may have noticed that I used the word "allow" in some of my instructions for non-verbal awareness. Part of doing this work involves allowing yourself to experience whatever you experience at the moment, accepting what you find.

People who work with me sometimes object that they want to change, not accept themselves as they presently function. However, as Gindler discovered, I find that people benefit from allowing themselves to experience whatever occurs. That doesn't mean you have to like what you experience. Nonetheless, positive changes can occur more easily when you're not denying or fighting what you experience. To control what you want to control, you have to experience it first.

My dear friend and teacher Charlotte Schuchardt Read has expressed this attitude beautifully in an interview on her sensory awareness work:

> This involves getting in touch with ourselves, and accepting what goes on. It's so important, I feel, to accept—not to criticize—ourselves, as in: "Oh! I shouldn't do this! I shouldn't do that!" But to accept what goes on. We all have built up habits over the years and we all could function a little better than we do. But to allow what we feel is needed —this is a big thing, you know. It really is so fundamental, at least in my view. Do we need more air? Do we need more keen observation? Do we need more silence? Oh, that's another important aspect of it, isn't it? To be able to be quiet.[6]

For example, I have used this approach for foot and leg cramps. I find that when I allow myself to focus on the sensations, noticing with interest (and varying degrees of difficulty) *how* the 'pain' feels, *how* the muscles twist…the cramp often disappears.

The Wedge of Awareness

Perhaps in reading this you have become a little more aware of your awareness. Your nervous system gives you the power to do this—the power of self-reflexiveness. Self-reflexiveness allows you actively to bring awareness to what was previously out of awareness. In this section I will show you how to apply the *Wedge of Awareness*, developed by General Semantics teacher Milton Dawes, to make practical use of this self-reflexive ability in order to improve your body awareness and posture-movement habits.[7]

Self-reflexiveness refers to the fact that you can make a map of a map. You can make a statement about a statement. This self-reflexive characteristic of our language reflects the underlying self-reflexive characteristic of our nervous systems, the ability to be conscious of our consciousness.

Whenever you find that an experience has stopped you short, you have made use of this self-reflexive capacity. For example, you've probably at some time in your life made a mis-step going down stairs because you 'thought' that there was another step to go down when there wasn't. Until the mis-step happened, you weren't aware that you had assumed that there was another step. This "oops" moment gave you a bit of unintentional awareness. You became aware of your level of awareness.

This kind of moment can begin to bring an aspect of choice into where you give your attention. It can lead to the practice of *intentional awareness*. Imagine yourself in the dark in an unfamiliar house, unable to find the light switch and having to go down some stairs. At such a time, as you carefully feel your way step by step, you may experience the kind of active, alert awareness that I refer to here. With intentional awareness, you make a deliberate decision to experience something specific and your attention is very much alive, awake and alert.

A wedge shape seems like an especially good symbol for such a moment of awareness. A wedge, like the kind that holds a door open, has a small edge through which it initially acts. This tiny tip gives it an effective point of action that allows the wedge to fit between the door and the floor. Another example of a wedge, an ax, has a very narrow cutting edge, which serves as its effective point of action. When you become aware of the automatic, 'mindless' aspects of your behavior you give yourself a Wedge of Awareness (WOA), also called Wedge of Consciousness (WOC).

You deliberately can seek out such moments. For example, if you habitually wear your watch on one wrist as most people do, switch it to the other wrist and notice the effect. You'll probably find that you have many "oops" moments throughout the day.

You also can 'WOA' yourself when you bring some intentional wedges to your ongoing activities. By applying a 'thin wedge' of awareness to a task, you can set clear, doable goals, no matter how small, that can be done even in one brief moment, here and now.

Astronaut Story Musgrave, in an interview discussing his repair work on the Hubble Space Telescope 368 miles above the Earth, described how you can do this:

"I have these little interrupts [WOAs] and they go off all the time. I'm doing a space walk, and the interrupts say, 'Look at the Earth, the sky, or inward. What are you feeling right now? Listen to your body.' It's an attempt to be a total participant, and at the same time getting the job done."[8]

Instead of this brief, incremental method of becoming 'mindful', i.e., changing habits, etc., we often do the opposite by 'applying the blunt side of the wedge' to our goals and to ourselves. You may set grand goals for yourself and attempt to change many things at once. For example, you may decide to practice sensory awareness twenty-four hours a day. This kind of approach seldom works.

In order to improve your posture-movement habits, you need to become more aware of what you do and how you do it. You will do best by starting modestly, taking brief moments, wedges, to observe yourself in action. You can practice sensory awareness by noticing one thing, one moment at a time.

As you become more aware of your body use, you will become more aware of other aspects of your life and the world around you. This works in reverse as well. Giving yourself time to pause and look at the scene around you or to sense how you're breathing, gives you a way of wedging yourself that will enhance your ability to move.

Interestingly enough, you will find that wedging yourself over time has a cumulative effect. Just as the size of a large area can be found by adding its small incremental parts, you may find that controlling small increments of your attention may add up to whole new habits of sensing and moving.

Stop right now and notice what you are doing. Give yourself a moment or two to answer each of these questions — not verbally but by noticing what you sense and feel:

Where are you located in space?

Where are you in relation to the corners of the room you're in?

Are you sitting in a chair or on a couch?

Can you feel what you are sitting on?

Can you feel your feet on the floor?

Are you sitting erect or slumping or somewhere in between?

Are you holding your breath or are you letting your breath flow freely?

What movements do you feel related to your breathing?

Do you allow enough space for your breathing?

Do you notice any tensions or pains at the moment?

What would you need at this moment to feel more comfortable?

How much of the length of your spine can you experience?

What kind of difference have these questions made in how you feel right now? You can wedge yourself by asking yourself these kinds of 'sense-able' questions. They will help you live more 'mindfully' as you observe and improve your habits of body mechanics and use.

You may even find it useful to get a small rubber or wooden wedge to place on your desk, work area or other place where you can see it often. Whenever you look at or handle the wedge you can remember to make and take a wedge of awareness.

Awareness, Inhibition and Direction

F. M. Alexander employed two dimensions of awareness that are important to remember as you work on improving your body mechanics and use. He called these dimensions "inhibition" and "direction" (see the previous discussion in Chapter 4) and they can easily be understood in terms of the wedge of awareness.

As you may recall from his story of self-discovery, in Chapter 4, Alexander found that when he decided to do something habitual like reciting a sentence, he found it difficult to prevent his old habits of misuse. If he immediately began to do the action, he pulled his head back, etc. Initially he was not even aware that he was continuing with his old habits of tension and malposture.

At some point, watching himself in his mirrors, etc., he realized that, despite his best intentions, he was continuing to tense and shorten himself while speaking. At the moment that he became aware of this, he was functioning at the "oops" level of awareness.

He began to realize that, at the critical moment when he decided to speak, the habit of tensing, pulling his head back, etc., seemed to get set off automatically unless he consciously decided to pause and delay his action. He called this process of having the notion of doing something and then delaying or not doing it immediately, "inhibition."

Bringing even a momentary pause into the chain of decision-making provided what Alexander discovered to be a means of developing new and better habits of using himself in speaking and other activities. "Inhibition," in the way I am using it here, *does not* refer to repressing any aspect of your behavior. Rather, stopping and pausing allows a wedge of awareness to enter a situation. Inhibition, in this sense, constitutes a 'negative' dimension of awareness.

"Direction" is the term used in the Alexander Technique to refer to a 'positive' dimension of awareness. A direction consists of an internal instruction that you give yourself in terms of a result you want to perceive. A direction can be given with words or images or just an internal desire to experience something in a certain way.

Alexander studied the conditions of better use in his own body. He came to understand that when he actually allowed his "neck to be free, to allow the head to go forward and up, to allow the back to lengthen and widen" the loss of voice that he had habitually experienced didn't happen.

While inhibiting his old response to the idea of speaking, he would project directions for better use by actually saying those words to himself. He found that the words, when their meanings had become clear through non-verbal exploration, pointed his awareness towards better use.

Alexander found that the process of giving directions worked best if he didn't try to *do* the directions. In other words, he found that he also had to inhibit any immediate action to carry out the directions. Instead, when he became aware of anything he was doing, say tightening his neck, that seemed incompatible with a particular direction, such as 'freeing the neck', he could simply stop doing the undesired action.

Inhibiting and directing can be considered as two sides of a wedge of awareness. Pausing (inhibiting) allows time for projecting (directing) a new pattern in place of automatic behavior. Conversely, when you give directions, such as "Let my neck be free" you automatically insert a pause into your habitual way of doing things. This is Dewey's "thinking in activity," mentioned at the end of the last chapter.

This notion of the wedge of awareness has broad implications for all sorts of behavior besides body mechanics. Alexander and other thinkers, such as Feldenkrais, have suggested that our body use constitutes a 'pivot' of habit in general. It is an intriguing notion that focusing on body mechanics in this 'mindful' way may provide a useful basis for developing the skill of thinking in activity in other areas of life.

Learning how to apply the wedge of awareness (which includes inhibition and direction) in relation to your body mechanics involves developing a conscious control system that you can 'insert' into your more or less automatic sequences of actions in daily life. In terms of Perceptual Control Theory, you can gradually 'recalibrate' your body image towards a better standard of use. This standard becomes a conscious reference level that helps you to direct yourself in activity any time you choose.

Mapping the Body

The brain seems to store what we perceive as a system of internal cognitive maps that represent the experience of our bodies and external environments. These internal cognitive maps provide the checkpoints that we use to set our goals and achieve our purposes.[9]

The limits of our actions, including how well we use our bodies, depend on the quality of our internal maps. Yet no map is perfect. No map is identical to the territory it represents. This 'obvious' statement leads to the non-obvious truth that your body map is not the same as your body and can sometimes mislead you.

Neurologist Oliver Sacks, in his book *The Man Who Mistook His Wife for a Hat,* demonstrates this phenomenon clearly in the extreme cases of people with serious brain damage. After certain kinds of strokes, for example, people may not recognize that their arm or leg belongs to them.[10]

Even those of us with normal brains easily can misperceive our bodies. This is what Alexander discovered when he was trying to change his body use. Dr. Wilfred Barlow documented this also in a study of army recruits who were asked to stand up without pulling their heads backwards. The recruits largely reported that they succeeded, although independent observation found the reverse.[11]

A map also does not cover all of the territory. There is a great deal going on in the body that we never perceive. At any one time the limits of our body awareness are confined by our span of attention and our habitual perception. Nonetheless, practicing body awareness can help you purposefully extend the range and accuracy of your cognitive body map.

Alexander Technique teachers Bill and Barbara Conable have elaborated the notion of what they call "Body Mapping" in some detail. As they point out, just studying your own anatomy and learning the parts, their relations and movements more accurately can help you gain better control of your body use.

One useful way you can do this is to review Chapter 5, especially the section "A Personal Anatomy Tour." If you haven't already done so (or even if you have) look at the picture of the skeleton and find the parts of the body on yourself.

Other ways to begin to better map your body include: getting a full body massage, getting a foot massage, soaking in a jacuzzi, having a 'bodywork' session such as Rolfing, Body Harmony, Shiatsu, etc., and, of course, pursuing a course of posture-movement education, i.e., the Alexander Technique.

Sensory-Motor Amnesia

Our body maps are not static and unchanging. They continue to be built and to develop through the constant barrage of sensations from muscle, joint and touch receptors as we move and interact with other people and other aspects of our environments. There is evidence that we require movement, touch and other kinds of experience on an ongoing basis in order to maintain a healthy body image. As anthropologist Ashley Montagu wrote, "The raw sensation of touch as stimulus is vitally necessary for the physical survival of the organism..." [12]

When an area becomes injured, this incoming information may become limited. We can become protective of the part with guarding and bracing efforts. As a result of a drop in 'normal' sensation, your body map may develop a blank spot that can affect your movements and well being. Pioneer posture-movement educator Thomas Hanna referred to this blank spot as "sensory-motor amnesia." [13]

When a severe enough injury has occurred, this feeling of a blank or "dead" area has been found to correlate with reduced neural activity in the sensory cortex, which has been measured by evoked-potential studies of the brain. This can occur not only with brain or nerve damage but as a result of peripheral injuries as well.[14]

Oliver Sacks writes about this phenomenon in his book, *A Leg to Stand On,* which recounts his own experience with a severe injury. While hiking, he fell and completely tore the tendon attachment of the muscle that extended his left leg. As he wrote, even after it had been surgically repaired and given time to heal, "I had come to question the integrity, the very existence, of my leg…"[15]

Sacks recounts the extraordinary process he went through to begin to walk. At first he did not even feel that the leg he was moving was his own. He had developed a profound sense of "alienation" from his leg and his normal self-image. What had to get re-mapped were not only the injured leg but also the daily actions that the leg had been involved with and the very sense of self he had before his injury.[16]

Sacks found that the process of recovery came in jumps and starts, with a number of reversals. One thing that accelerated this process was the advice of a wise physician he consulted who asked, "What do you enjoy doing?" When Sacks replied that he loved to swim, the doctor made a phone call and immediately sent him over to a pool for a rehabilitative swim.

Sacks got to the pool, changed into trunks and hobbled with his cane to the side of the pool to meet the lifeguard who was expecting him. The young man challenged him to a race, grabbed the cane out of his hand and pushed him into the pool. After their race, Sacks stepped out of the pool and found that he was walking normally again. (This appears similar to the story of my wife's sprained foot, told in Chapter 10 in the section on Guarding and Movement Sensation.)

As Sacks describes it "...unexpectedness, spontaneity, somehow evoking a natural response, ...lay at the heart of [his doctor's] theory and practice of therapy — the finding of some activity which was natural and meaningful, an expression of a will that found delight in itself..." [17]

Can this sort of thing happen with injuries to the back? If you are recovering from a back or neck injury, this notion of 'sensory-motor amnesia' may have some relevance for you. If you find that you still are not functioning quite normally even if you are free or mostly free from pain, it may be useful to find what you really enjoy doing and start doing it.

For example, to encourage spontaneous movement, find some music with a good rhythm that you enjoy (I like Billy Idol's "Dancing With Myself"). Close the door and blinds so no one will see you (if you find dancing with yourself embarrassing) and move to the music. As you explore the possibilities of movement, stay attentive to your back so you can respond sensitively to feelings of comfort and discomfort. You can move as quickly or slowly, as much or as little as you feel comfortable doing. "There's nothing to lose and there's nothing to prove."[18] Let the music move you.

Enjoying this and some of the other bodily experiences mentioned in this chapter will help you begin to re-extend your body map and begin to feel your bodily self, beyond pain, as a source of happiness and enjoyment.

Chapter 13

Experience Your Full Stature

The second guideline for better body use is: *Experience your full stature every day as often as you can.*

In this chapter we explore what *full stature* means, what it *doesn't* mean, some 'recipes' for experiencing more of your full stature and some ways to begin experimenting with it in your daily life.

I have already noted the fallibility of our internal cognitive maps.[1] Our body maps *are not* our bodies. Our body maps *are not* complete and can always be revised and improved. These limitations must be faced if you wish to cultivate your use. They also prevent me from guaranteeing that you can achieve an *adequate* standard of use simply by reading this book.

Nonetheless, it is possible to improve on your own to some degree by 'wedging' yourself. These pages can provide the background you need for improving how you do this.

Full Stature - What It *Doesn't*—and *Does*—Mean

One of the major problems that people have with trying to improve their 'posture' involves trying to impose a static and unchanging map of body use on themselves and others. "Sitting up or standing up straight" gets translated into the action of holding yourself in a stiff and unyielding way.

What happens when people try to 'fix themselves up' by holding such stiff and rigid postures? Not only doesn't it work very well—it also imposes another layer of misuse on the body. Think of an army recruit standing rigidly at attention: shoulders pulled back; chest puffed out; back arched in a hyperextended pose; knees locked; etc. That is not what I mean by "full stature."

Instead, full stature implies the total volume or space of your body. Practically, this involves keeping all your joints as open and unlocked as possible, with plenty of factor-of-safety motion present.

Because of the mechanical linkages of all of the parts, this is more likely to happen when you *allow your spine, the central axis of your body, to lengthen within its natural curves.* When you are lengthening your spine in this way, your anti-gravity system works at its best. You are encouraging what Goddard Binkley, a teacher of the Alexander Technique, called "the expanding self"[2] and are ready for dealing with the world.

Imposition of a rigid standard on yourself can happen even if you intellectually understand what good use entails. It occurs especially if you assume that you can automatically apply your understanding to your non-verbal actions.

Rather, full stature needs to be something that you experience non-verbally. When you have developed an adequate internal standard, a non-verbal map of full stature, you can direct yourself to better use without holding or trying.

Viewing the rules of good use as rigid and inflexible has some relation to a rigid and inflexible manner of holding yourself. In my teaching, I work at helping people establish better use without absolute rules.

It does not seem realistic to expect anyone to be lengthened at his or her full stature 100% of the time. If you use yourself well 75% of the time, your use will probably be better than 98% of the population. Full stature is a standard that you can apply to your postural behavior, while knowing that no cosmic law says that you cannot slouch. So by all means *slouch whenever you want to.* Slouch consciously when you do and become aware of the results.

My basic guideline remains *choice.* Realize that when you have the ability to choose how you use yourself you have more of a chance to control pain and to move with more grace and efficiency. But by all means don't 'should' on yourself.

Constructive Rest

Constructive rest is a term used by Lulu Sweigard, a writer on body mechanics whose work parallels the Alexander Technique.[3] I like the term "constructive rest" because it emphasizes the possibility of actively restoring yourself during your waking hours. A constructive rest position places the body so that gravity assists in releasing the muscles and opening the joints to help you experience more of your full stature.

Spending from ten to twenty minutes in constructive rest once or twice a day will give you an opportunity to give yourself space, both figuratively and literally. When you feel yourself in a slump and having trouble holding yourself up, even five minutes of constructive rest can help you restore yourself.

Here, in summary, is a simple and effective constructive rest position. I discuss details in the following paragraphs. Lie on your back on a firm surface, with your knees bent and feet 'standing' apart, so that your legs can balance with no muscular effort. Your body will be lying symmetrically with equal parts on either side of an imaginary line through your midsection and in line with your spine. Your head will rest on enough books so that it is not tilted backwards on your neck. The front of your neck as well as the back of your neck should lie relaxed and open. Your head should neither be unduly protruded (pushed forward) nor overly retracted (shifted back). Ideally, the top of your head is directed in an imaginary line away from your tailbone (see Figure 13.1).

In this position, the curves of your lower back and neck will be reduced and will approximate a straight line. Do not try to force your lower back or neck 'straight'. If you have found benefit in extending your lower back, you can place a small towel roll or other support under your lumbar spine to support the curve, which can reduce pressure on your discs.

Your arms can be positioned to rest at your sides in such a way that they are easily supported on the surface you are lying on. They can also be placed so that your hands rest over the front of your torso on your belly. The important thing here is minimum effort.

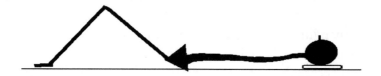

Figure 13.1 — A Constructive Rest Position

For your lying down surface, a carpeted floor or a wooden floor covered with a blanket will be fine. A firm surface that feels comfortable and that allows you to sense your back is most desirable. Make sure that you are warm enough and have a sheet, blanket or afghan available to cover yourself with if necessary. Have four or five paperback books ready to supply head support. You may have to experiment with different numbers of books. You can place them where you plan to rest your head. The 'give' of the books should also have a balance of firmness and comfort. If the back of your head feels sensitive put a small cloth or layer of foam on top of the book on which you rest.

There are many ways to get yourself into your constructive rest position. Whatever method you choose, take time to pay attention to the process by which you bring yourself to the floor. Stay with yourself and with lengthening your spine as you do this.

Once you are lying down, use enough books under your head so that the length of your neck is as unimpaired as possible, both in the back and front. The ideal is just a sufficient number of books for your head not to be tilted backwards. If parts of your neck seem stiff, do the best you can. Don't force anything. Support the back of your head with one or both hands when you lift it in order to avoid any sense of straining, when, for example, adding or removing books.

If you are lying down on your back with your legs out straight, you will need to bring your knees up in order to balance them and also to help your back release. As you bring up your knees, continue to breathe normally and continue to free your neck. Don't tighten it or your back.

The thought of your legs lengthening out from your pelvis, knees releasing away from your hip sockets, will help you to keep the joints of your legs open and released. Let your feet come as close to your buttocks as possible without strain and far enough apart from one another to allow you to release the muscles around your hips and buttocks. Your legs eventually should be able to balance without any muscular effort.

You may want to gently lift your bottom up from the floor so that your pelvis and part of your lower back is raised. Then gently let your back and buttocks return to the floor. You may feel at this point that your back is making more contact with the floor. In this horizontal position, the curves will not necessarily need to be as accentuated. But don't try to force them flat.

I like to encourage people to use a lumbar support if they can. If you want to use a towel roll or other lumbar support, place it under your back when you lift up. I particularly like to use the Spinatrac™ posture tool, a gentle curve made of firm plastic that feels comfortable and unobtrusive.[4]

Another adjustment you can make is to 'iron out' your upper back. To do this gently, reach one hand towards the ceiling and slightly across the midline to the opposite side. Do this with the thought of lengthening your arm from shoulder to fingertips. As you do this, notice that your shoulder blade can gently release away from your spine. Gently let your arm settle back down. You can do the same with your opposite hand and shoulder blade.

Once you have gotten yourself into this constructive rest position, you can bring your awareness to your full length and width by repeating your directions to yourself. This provides a good way of scanning your body for tensions and allowing them to release. You can actually say the words to yourself:

• Let my neck free...

• To let my head go forwards and up...

• To let my back lengthen and widen...

• To let my shoulders release apart from each other...

• To let my arms lengthen and release from my shoulder to elbow to wrist and hand and out my finger tips...

• To let my legs release from my pelvis...lengthening from my hips to my knees...knees to ankles... from my heels to my toes...

When you want to get up from constructive rest, take enough time to keep the awareness of lengthening, widening and releasing that you now have. Roll onto your side and continue with thoughts of lengthening up along your spine. To get yourself up you can come onto your side...onto hands and knees...onto one knee...and up to standing, using a chair for support if you need it. Feel what it's like standing again. Walk around a bit. How do you feel? How can you continue to lengthen and widen, as you remain up and about?

Sitting 'Up'

If you want to sit for longer periods with less chance of irritating your back, you will need to learn how to sit 'up' — to support yourself at your full stature when sitting. When sitting at full stature, you will be lengthening throughout your spine while maintaining its normal curves.

Your neck will be releasing and lengthening to allow your head to balance forwards and up on top of your lengthening spine. Meanwhile your back and torso will be lengthening and widening. The joints of your spine will have sufficient factor-of-safety motion. They will not be positioned at end range. In order for this to occur, your postural muscles, including your deep spinal extensors and abdominal muscles, will have to engage sufficiently to support this lengthened stature.

Instead, as we have seen, exactly the opposite typically happens—the seated slump wherein the back is at the extreme of flexion, with the joints at end range and hanging on over-stretched spinal ligaments. In this slump, your postural muscles are not 'asked' to work and they don't.

People often ask me what type of chair is best for them to use. Some types of chairs and seat designs do seem more mechanically advantageous. However, depending on chairs for support often doesn't work. No chair is perfect. Chairs are often designed more for visual aesthetics than for better body mechanics. Shaping our bodies to such questionable seating leads to collapse and strain rather than true support.[5]

My best advice is to learn how to sit at your full stature supported and unsupported. This will help you develop a standard by which to judge which chairs and seats help you to do this better. Here I will provide you with some simple ways to begin to work on your own to learn better sitting with and without a back support.

A useful chair for practicing sitting is a simple kitchen or dining room chair with a back. The seat height should allow your knees to go no higher than hip joint level. In fact, having your knees a bit lower than your hips can facilitate a more neutral position for your back and legs. You can achieve this with a wedge cushion, for example, which creates a forward sloping seat (there are even special chairs that do this).[6] Your seat should allow you to let your feet rest easily on the floor. The seat depth, its distance from front edge to chair back, should support your thighs without digging into the backs of your knees when you sit against the chair back.

Supported Sitting

To sit using the back of the chair, scoot your bottom all the way back until you feel the base of your spine against the chair back. You should be able to feel the mid-parts of your sit bones on the seat below you. If you lack sufficient built-in 'padding' of your own make sure the seat has enough for comfort. Now you will be able to let your back's full length and width rest against the chair's back support, which ideally will come up to shoulder level.

There has been some controversy about the use of lumbar supports. Although there may be occasional exceptions, in general I agree with Cyriax, who wrote as early as 1945 about the importance of maintaining the lumbar lordosis when sitting.[7] Maintaining the lordosis has been advocated by some medical doctors for more than a century as a vital part of good sitting posture.[8] Maintaining a sitting lordosis probably has importance for you.

A lumbar roll can help you to do this. Sitting with a lumbar roll has been shown to help reduce symptoms in patients with sciatica.[9] It's important to be able to adjust the size and position of the support. Built-in supports don't adjust as easily as portable rolls. You will probably do better with a simple portable roll that you can move from chair to chair. Even a rolled-up towel can work in a pinch. The support should be placed at the level of your lower lumbar area and should "conform with the curve" there.[10] Even as you sit with your support, remember to direct yourself to let your neck release to allow your head to balance up on top of your lengthening spine. You will need to work to ensure that you don't protrude your head and neck.

Sitting supported by a chair back is not as demanding on the postural muscles as unsupported sitting. It will be a useful position to sit in for brief periods if you are just getting back to sitting after a back injury.

There is a major disadvantage in sitting against a chair back with a lumbar support. When you are sitting and working or eating, etc., you are not likely to stay still. As soon as you move, you will no longer have the external support. So you need to know how to sit with your full stature unsupported.

Unsupported Sitting

Unsupported sitting means no outside support. Instead, you will be sitting with good internal support from your own postural mechanisms, that is, your anti-gravity muscles, discs, etc. You can begin to get a feel for sitting up unsupported by experimenting with what McKenzie calls "the slouch over-correct" maneuver.[11]

This is an advanced 'exercise' to be done when you have recovered from an acute episode of back pain. View it as an experiment primarily for your awareness. It is based on the principle that sometimes by experiencing the extremes of a condition, you can begin to recognize where the 'golden mean' (desirable neutral state) exists.

To perform this maneuver, slide yourself away from the back support so you are sitting near the edge of the chair, feet on the floor. Feel where your sit bones are making contact with the chair. Think of your sit bones as the 'feet of the pelvis' and find out where the mid-point of these 'feet' are located.

Now, roll backwards with your whole pelvis so that you go back towards the 'heels' of your sit bones. Then roll further so that you are beginning to sit on your tailbone. As you do this, your lower back will begin to lose its lordosis, then flatten until it is in full flexion. If you continue to face and look forwards, this maneuver with your pelvis will automatically cause your head and neck to protrude in front of your body as your head tilts backwards on your neck. You will be in a maximally slumped position. This is the "slouch" phase depicted on the left of Figure 13.2.

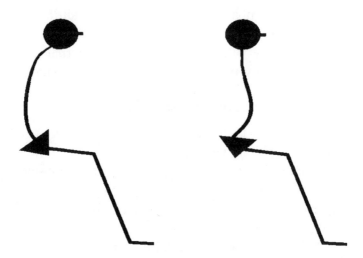

Figure 13.2 — "Slouch Overcorrect" Maneuver

Next comes the "overcorrect" phase depicted on the right side of Figure 13.2. Continuing to face and look forwards, roll your pelvis forwards so that you are moving towards the 'toes' of your sit bones. Go as far as you can so that you feel as if you are beginning to sit more on your thighs. Your lower back will extend into an exaggerated lordosis or hollow arch. If you continue to face and look forwards you will notice that your spine will lengthen a bit as the back of your head rolls forwards in relation to your upper neck and your head and neck will be in relative retraction (pulled back over your body) from its previous protruded position. If you feel a strain in your lower back you are probably in the fully arched or overcorrected position. We call this "overcorrected" because it exaggerates a 'good', neutral, sitting posture.

Now let yourself return to the previous slouched position. Go back and forth between the slouched and the overcorrected positions. You can do this five to ten times. Get a feel for the change in the overall shape of your spine. Notice what effect the two extremes have on your relative height, on your breathing, etc.

With the last overcorrected movement that you make, ease out of it about 10 to 15%, so that you feel you are about at 'neutral'. Your weight will be centered over the mid-portion of your sit bones. Your back will be slightly, not exaggeratedly, arched. Think of freeing your neck, of your head balancing up on top of your spine, your back and torso lengthening and widening. Remember to allow yourself to breathe. This balanced, neutral sitting posture is depicted in Figure 13.3.

McKenzie recommends doing five to fifteen repetitions of this maneuver, three times a day, for three to four days or longer.[12] It may take at least several weeks for balanced sitting to become habitual.

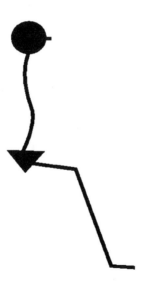

Figure 13.3 — Balanced Neutral Sitting

When you are familiar with the mid-position of balanced neutral sitting, you can also begin to practice building your sitting endurance. You gradually can extend your unsupported sitting to longer periods of time as you become more comfortable with it and as your muscles and joints become more adjusted. Working in this way, you will begin to train yourself to sit 'up' with your full stature.

Leaning Forwards in the Chair

Direct your attention to the changes in the position of your head, neck and upper back that you've just experienced. The protrusion of your head and neck in the slouched position is often the actual starting point of an active slouch in daily life because of the desire to bend forwards or to see better what's in front of you. Done frequently, this can lead to an habitual protruded head and the familiar "dowager's hump."

In order to avoid this habitual distortion of your body, you need to learn how to move your whole torso as a unit when you lean forwards. As Ron Dennis, Ed.D., founder of PostureSense®, says, "Fold, don't bend your body."[13] This applies both when you sit and stand. Later, I will discuss how to apply this while standing. Now, you can take yourself through the steps of doing this while sitting.

Sitting to the best of your ability with your full stature, think of leaning forwards by coming up and over your hip joints with your whole torso lengthening. Pause (inhibit) before actually carrying out this movement. Then give yourself these directions: "Let my neck stay free, to let my head balance up on top of my lengthening spine, to let my back lengthen and widen." Then you can stay with this sense of length up through your spine as you let yourself flex at your hip creases.

If you are actually doing this you will roll forward over your sit bones. As illustrated in Figure 13.4, your head, neck and back will remain in a constant relation with each other as they fold up and over as a unit at the hip joints. Doing this in front of a mirror can help you to make sure you are actually doing what you think you are doing.

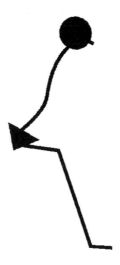

Figure 13.4 – Folding In Sitting

Standing With Poise

Poise implies not only a certain manner of bodily use but also a certain psychological attitude, one of composure, calm and presence of 'mind'. This connection between bodily attitude and 'mental' attitude only seems like an interesting co-incidence because of the persistent separation of 'body' and 'mind' in our culture. In fact, since what we separate as 'body' and 'mind' actually involves an organism–as–a–whole–in–an–environment, bodily use will necessarily have 'mental', emotional aspects.

Learning how to stand with poise at your full stature will help you to function more comfortably when standing. It can also help you become more calm and present in any situation.

This seems especially important when you find yourself in front of others, for example, while giving a presentation. Below I present some basic guidance for helping you explore "active, alerted"[14] standing at your full stature.

There is a range of possible ways to slump while standing.[15] The weight is often shifted towards the balls of the feet. The knees will often be locked in hyperextension. The pelvis may be shifted forwards as the person hangs with the hip joints locked in extension. The lumbar spine curve may appear either at the extreme end range of hyperextension or flattened and even flexed in the opposite direction. The rest of the spine will often be shortened in some degree of collapse, with the head and neck protruded. The head may tilt backwards on the upper neck while the upper back forms a flexed hump.

To explore your own standing, stand up. Without trying to change anything, notice if you can observe any of the factors mentioned in the previous paragraph or anything else that seems especially prominent. When you notice a 'fault', congratulate yourself, since you have noticed something that you didn't notice before. This provides you with a potential wedge of awareness that can lead to positive change.

Exploring Your Base of Support

Begin to explore your base of support.[16] Do this with your shoes off. Spread your legs apart so that your feet are approximately shoulder width apart. Let your toes point gently forwards and perhaps a bit outwards to the sides. See if you can allow your kneecaps to point in the same direction as your toes without forcing.

Let your knees be easy and unlocked (that doesn't mean bending them appreciably but rather not holding them stiffly in full extension). Begin to notice where your weight is distributed over your feet. Do you feel more weight over one foot? Where on your feet do you feel most of your weight, towards the toes, heels or throughout the whole foot? Perhaps one foot feels different than the other.

Think the directions of "letting my neck release to let my head balance up on top of my lengthening spine" as you gently let your whole body move over your ankle joints to come forwards towards the balls of your feet. As you do so, don't lose your balance or let your heels raise. The movement will be small. Then shift backwards towards your heels without losing balance or letting your toes raise up. Remember to keep your knees unlocked. Continue to direct your whole spine into length while you free your neck.

If you don't feel secure about your balance while doing this, stand with your back to a wall or a chair and with something like a chair or shelf in front or to the side that you can hold onto.

Now shift forwards and backwards again, towards the balls, then the heels of your feet. After about ten or so repetitions of this, let your weight come to rest near your heels. To find where your weight is most evenly balanced on your feet, shift slightly forwards. This is likely to be somewhat closer to your heels than you are used to. Think of your whole foot lengthening and widening as it makes contact with the ground. Remember to keep your knees easy and unlocked. Place the tips of your fingers along your groin crease and gently direct your hip joints to unlock and stay back. Think of lengthening up along your spine, your head balancing up on top of your spine.

If you have been able to follow these instructions accurately, you will find yourself in a basic balanced stance that permits more of your full stature. It does seem that the head, neck and back lead the rest of the body into length. However, in a circular fashion, finding greater balance in your base of support seems to provide the necessary foundation for your head, neck and back to lead you.

Weight–Shifting for Side-to-Side Balance

There are other experiments you can do to explore and enhance your standing stature, to stand with poise. For example, with feet shoulder-width apart and knees and hips unlocked, let your neck release your head to balance up on top of your spine as you lengthen and widen your back. As you continue lengthening up, let your whole body shift fully onto your right foot without lifting your left from the floor. Then shift over to your left foot. Go back and forth so that you are weight–shifting right and left five to ten times. Go slowly enough to experience what is happening in yourself while you do it. Make sure you don't poke your 'hips' out to the side. Keep your trunk level (don't bend to the side) and keep your knees as easy and unlocked as possible.

The purpose of both the front-to-back and side-to-side experiments is to help you get a greater sense of your possibilities of balance in standing. The most balanced standing involves an unstable equilibrium where your joints are unlocked (with a factor-of-safety present) and your muscles are ready to 'kick in' automatically when needed. When you are standing with this kind of balance, you will be standing 'still' but will be able to allow continuing movement.

I want to emphasize here that in standing there is no one correct way to position your feet. In asking you to do the above experiments with your feet standing side by side, I don't want you to infer that you 'should' necessarily always stand like that in your everyday activities, though you sometimes can. Your choices are many. For example, you can find a comfortable and balanced way of standing by having one foot slightly in front of the other with your weight mostly on the back foot. However you choose to stand, continue with a few wedges of awareness to release, lengthen, widen.

Standing with Your Center

I once gave some Alexander Technique lessons to an acupuncturist who told me that it seemed to him we were doing a form of Qigong [pronounced chee gung], "energy healing" in Chinese.[17] I later discovered a Chinese term that seems especially related to the 'mindful' body mechanics I teach. The term "diao shen" stands for "regulating the body."[18]

As I've explored this area, I've discovered that Eastern traditions of martial, meditative, movement and healing arts, like Tai Chi Chuan, Zen, Qigong and Yoga, share some connections with what I've been presenting here. One does not need to adhere to traditional Oriental medical theory to acknowledge useful aspects of these practical arts. Among these useful aspects is an emphasis on the importance of posture.

Kenneth S. Cohen, in his book *The Way of Qigong*, summarizes traditional Chinese advice on posture that correlates closely with more modern systems of teaching about body mechanics, such as the Alexander Technique:

> …when practicing qigong, keep in mind the following: relax the whole body, especially the joints; keep the neck relaxed and the head suspended delicately over the spine; the jaw is also relaxed, with the tongue generally touching the upper palate; sink the shoulders and elbows; maintain a relaxed but erect spine, centered and stable; maximize contact between the feet and the ground, feeling your body's weight dropping *through* the feet; release the sternum; the spine is long and extended; the hips are relaxed. Do not use force! Be aware of what you are doing! The abdomen is relaxed, and the breath feels as though it is sinking into it.[19]

This last instruction deserves special attention. The level of the lower abdomen (where the center of gravity is located in standing) is called the "dan tian" in Chinese, "hara" in Japanese. Philosopher and psychotherapist Karlfried Graf Von Dürkheim called this "the vital centre of man [and woman]." Martial artists advise one to "sink the qi or ki [hypothetical vital 'energy'] to the dan tian or hara."

In practice, this involves bringing your awareness of breath-related movement into your center and releasing any needless tensions there. As you do this you can imagine your breath as a white light or 'energy' going into the area (use of such imagery may help you direct your awareness better even as you realize that what you imagine may not be happening in the way you imagine it).

To get a better sense of your center, stand and place one hand palm down over your belly just below your navel. Place the back of your other hand behind your back between the lumbar and sacral levels so it comes even with your front hand. Imagine the midpoint between your hands. Without forcing anything, think about the movement related to your breath coming into the area between your hands. As you continue, you may be able to feel your hands move with your breathing. As you feel more of the movement of your breath in your lower abdomen and back, locate the place where your breath seems to be expanding from inside yourself. Notice any other movements in your chest, abdomen and back related to your breathing.

Awareness of your center area can improve your sense of connection between your legs and torso and thus enhance your balance and support in standing. Therefore, in addition to the basic Alexander Technique directions, you may benefit by adding attention to your center:

• Free your neck...

- To allow your head to balance forwards and up on top of your spine...

- To allow your back (torso) to lengthen and widen...

- As you bring awareness and breath to your center...

- Etc...

Here is another experiment to bring a sense of your center into standing and balancing. It involves imagining a pencil-thin laser beam that originates in your center and flows up through the length of your body and out the top of your head. With each part of the exercise, you can imagine the path the laser beam takes on the ceiling related to the path in which you are moving.

Gently bring your hands over the center area with one hand on your lower belly and the other on your lower back. As you free your neck, let your head balance up on top of your spine by imagining that your head is suspended from above by a string like a marionette. Let this thought help you to lengthen up along your spine. With awareness of your head balancing, and of your center, move your feet shoulder width apart. Imagine the pencil-thin laser beam flowing up from your center and through the length of your body and out the top of your head.

Then, keeping your hands over your center or allowing them to hang at your side, begin to let your weight shift from one foot to the other as you did in the previous side-to-side experiment. Imagine the laser beam making a horizontal line as it meets the ceiling while you shift side to side. Be aware of how your center point moves along that same line. Continue shifting five to ten times.

Now slightly shift your weight forwards and backwards, toes to heels and back again. Don't put yourself off balance.

You can continue with your hands over your center if you wish. Imagine that the laser beam from your center goes out the top of your head and makes a vertical line on the ceiling. In your imagination, see how your center point is also moving along that vertical line. Do this five to ten times.

Now shift over the base of support of your feet in a clockwise circle so that the imaginary laser beam from your center forms a clockwise circle on the ceiling as it goes out the top of your head. Remember to free your neck and to breathe. After five to ten times clockwise, go in the opposite direction so that the imaginary circle on the ceiling will be going counterclockwise. With each of these movements your weight will be shifting over your feet to the side, back, other side, front, again to the side, etc.

You also can do the above exercises while focusing your attention on the movement of your center over the base of support of your feet or on the shifting pressures in your feet themselves. Once you coordinate yourself while doing these movements, you will be balancing yourself with whole body awareness in head, center and feet. After you stop, stand quietly, then walk around a bit. Notice how you feel.

Practicing such 'mindful' experiments in standing balance will make it easier to apply a wedge of awareness to yourself, whether you are standing in a line or in front of a group giving a presentation. You can also bring this awareness to your walking. When you walk you can bring your awareness to the shifting of weight over your feet, to the movement of your center, to how your head balances, etc.

Full Stature for Full Breathing and Vice Versa

F. M. Alexander was known as "the breathing man" when he first developed his work in Australia.[20] Both he and his students became aware that, when they functioned more often at their full stature, their breathing tended to improve as well.

Other workers in the field of body mechanics have noted the relation of breathing and posture. Goldthwait explained how the drooping chest that accompanies a chronically flexed spine reduces the factor-of-safety motion in the ribs. By keeping the points of connection of the abdominal muscles and the diaphragm too close together, it also interferes with the optimal action of these 'breathing' muscles.[21]

Research by John H. M. Austin, M.D., and Pearl Ausubel indicates that people who have had Alexander Technique lessons show significant improvement in some respiratory function measurements compared to those who have not had lessons.[22] This has obvious relevance for singers, actors and many musicians whose work directly depends on their breath. Perhaps that explains in part why people from these professions have been among the most eager students of the 'mindful' mechanics of the Alexander Technique.

Even if you're not a singer (except in the shower) or an actor (except on the 'stage' of life), this has relevance for you. By exploring the relation of your breathing and stature on your own, you can begin to benefit from the wedges of awareness you gain.

Start by bringing yourself into a slump either sitting or standing. Let your head protrude as far as possible in front of your body, head tilting backwards on your neck, back collapsed, etc. (I hope that this has begun to feel unpleasant!) Notice how much space you have in your neck, torso and abdomen. Bring your attention to your breathing. What movements can you sense in relation to your breathing?

Now free your neck and let it move back over your spine without straining as you allow your head to tilt forwards (in relation to your upper neck). As you do this your head will also move up to balance on top your spine, leading the rest of your body up into greater length. Allow your spine to lengthen, your back and torso to lengthen and widen, etc. Make sure you're not holding or tensing unnecessarily to do this. Notice how much space you're allowing yourself now. Bring your attention to your breathing once again. What movements do you now sense in relation to your breathing?

By becoming more aware of the differences between these two extremes of posture, you can enhance both your stature and your breathing. By lengthening and widening your torso to approach your full stature, you will be allowing the optimal space for your breathing. In turn, making sure that you are allowing your breathing and the natural movements related to it ensures that you are not tensing your postural muscles with unnecessary effort.

In the previous section, I described a way of enhancing the space for breathing by locating your center area with your hands and letting this area release as you let the movement related to your breathing come into it.

Another method for enhancing your breathing consists of a procedure from the Alexander Technique known as *The Whispered Ah*.[23] This procedure works as a set of guidelines for becoming aware of different aspects of your use that go into your breathing and voice. It also provides a means of stimulating your breathing and voice.

The Whispered Ah is done in a stepwise fashion, with awareness given at each step to freeing your neck, lengthening up along your spine, etc. The steps:

1. Direct your neck free, to allow your head to balance forwards and up on top of your spine, to allow your back and torso to lengthen and widen.

2. Let the tip of your tongue go behind your lower teeth (lips remain gently closed, teeth apart).

3. Let a smile come to your face by thinking of something amusing. If you can't think of anything that makes you smile, fake it! There you go.

4. Notice your breath going in (inhalation) and out (exhalation). When you have a sense of the rhythm of your breathing...

5. Exhale through your mouth with a whispered and audible "Ahhhh" as you let your mouth open (your tongue pointing your jaw forwards as you let your jaw release open).

6. At the end of this easy exhalation of "Ah," let your lips gently close as you allow air to come in through your nose.

That is the end of a single cycle of the Whispered Ah. You can then return to step 1 and repeat the cycle five or six times.

As you follow the steps you will realize that there are a lot of things to keep track of. Remember especially not to prepare for step 5 by trying to take in a breath. Let the "Ah" come as a result of the previous inhalation. One of the things that you can discover doing the Whispered Ah is that what many people do to take in a deep breath, that is, actively inhaling by sucking in or gasping for a breath, is not necessary. The inhalation will take care of itself after you fully exhale. You can let the inhalation happen.

The Whispered Ah can also help you become aware of the movements in your ribs and abdomen and of the possibilities for releasing your face and jaw. It provides a good warm-up that you can do prior to singing or speaking or at any other time that you want to enhance your breathing.

Dynamic Use in Standing

There is a danger that my written descriptions here have appeared to emphasize static 'posture' at the expense of dynamic use. This dynamic aspect is difficult to convey in print. So I want to emphasize that functioning with a more full stature is *not* about becoming a more full 'statue'.

The Alexander Technique distinguishes itself as a form of body mechanics training because of its emphasis on *dynamic* posture or *use within movement*. Beckett Howorth, M.D., defined dynamic posture as

> ...posture in motion or in action or in preparation for action. It includes the transitions between the static positions...and also activities such as pushing, lifting... [etc.]...Good dynamic posture implies the use of the body or its parts in the simplest and most effective way, using muscle contraction and relaxation, balance, coordination, rhythm and timing as well as gravity, inertia and momentum to optimum advantage. The smooth integration of these elements of good dynamic posture results in neuromusculoskeletal performance which is easy, graceful, satisfying and effective and represents the best in the individual physical activity, as well as in the physical activity of the individual.[24]

Because of this dynamic element, the suggestions that I give here can provide you with only the bare beginnings for better use. Static words cannot necessarily give you the same kind of dynamic experience that you get in a PostureSense® class or in an Alexander Technique lesson. Both involve varying degrees of verbal and manual guidance by a teacher as you perform different activities of daily living.[25]

Another danger when following these or any other suggestions involves not spending enough time observing yourself before trying to change things. I urge you *not* to hurry to fix yourself. Instead *use the suggestions in this book as starting points for body awareness and self-observation.* The efforts you make to observe yourself more closely in your everyday activities will result in more substantial improvement than if you immediately try to move with 'perfect' posture.

You need to taste, chew and digest whatever suggestions I give you so that you can apply what you find useful for yourself. Trying to 'be right' may only mean that you are 'swallowing whole' what I say here without 'chewing' it sufficiently for yourself. You can explore for yourself what works and what doesn't work, using my suggestions as guidelines. This can be a cyclic or, rather, a spiral process — starting with a picture of your desired goals for better movement; self-observation while moving; revised goals; self-correction; etc. The resulting knowledge of better use will be your own.

Let's apply this attitude of observing and spiraling self-improvement to an action we do every day: bending forwards. Bending activities may include bending at the sink, bending to pick something up from the floor, shoveling snow, vacuuming, sweeping, lifting, etc.

Our eyes are located in the front of our heads (though my wife also seems to have eyes in the back of her head!) and our hands work more easily in front than behind. This means that we often lower ourselves in order to deal with some aspect of the environment located in front of and below us. We may also bend forwards in standing up and in lowering ourselves to sit down.

Bending is often a troublesome action for those with back pain. Indeed, acute episodes of mechanical back pain often begin with a forward-bending motion. What typically happens to your stature when bending the way that you usually do?

Start with some self-observation. You may decide, for example, to notice what happens to your stature—the relations among your head, neck and torso—when you wash your hands at the sink. You can pick this as something to observe for the day. Initially, don't try to change anything. Simply find out what you are doing. (Simple is not necessarily easy!)

At first you may find that you already have bent over before you remember that you intended to observe yourself. That's okay—it's a wedge of awareness. Just remind yourself to observe yourself the next time you bend over at the sink.

What do you observe when you go to bend over?

Do you protrude your head and neck?

Do you find that your head gets tilted backwards or forwards on top of your neck?

To what degree does this happen?

What is the overall shape of your spine and torso?

Is your upper or lower back rounded into flexion?

How much do you flex at the hip joints?

Do you flex your knees at all?

How are you balancing yourself?

Do you feel strain, tension or pain anywhere?

What happens to your breathing?

It may take some time to get more of a sense of what you actually do. Using a mirror or mirrors to see a forward and side view, as Alexander did, can help you get a more accurate picture of yourself as you bend. Getting a friend or other outside observer can often help as well.

Folding in Standing

The idea of bending may have become so connected with losing your full stature that you may find it more helpful, as Ron Dennis suggests, to think about folding rather than bending your body.[26] This has also been called squatting. It involves lowering and raising your center of gravity, while maintaining your full stature and balance over your feet, while folding at your hips, knees and ankles in varying degrees. Discovering how to fold to maintain more of your full stature can result in greater efficiency and reduced injury. A mirror can help as you take yourself through the next phase of dynamic use to practice folding rather than bending while standing.

Start with no concern at all for any practical activity like lowering yourself to the sink; you are simply experiencing yourself moving. Begin by bringing yourself to full and balanced standing. Free your neck; let your head balance up on top of your spine as if suspended from the top of your head. Allow your spine to lengthen in its curves as you let your back lengthen and widen, your torso lengthen and widen. Let your breast bone drop as you let your spine lengthen. You can bring your legs wide apart with your feet pointing forwards and knees unlocked. Let your hips stay back. Bring your attention to the center area of your lower abdomen and pelvis.

Think of folding rather than bending, and pause—don't do it yet! (a moment of inhibition). *Think* of yourself getting drawn upwards from the crown of your head as you continue to lengthen your spine. Then let your knees fold, letting them move gently over your feet as you think of them releasing away from your hip joints.

At first just let your knees and hips fold just enough so that your center, the center of gravity of your body, sinks slightly lower while your spine and torso stay vertical. You won't necessarily be folding your knees very far. Do not force anything.

Pause and return to the directions of releasing your neck, letting your head go out from the top of your spine as your spine lengthens. Then let your hip joints release back as you let your knees fold more. You may find that your torso has begun to incline forward. Let your arms hang freely from your shoulders. You will find yourself in a mini-squat, as seen in Figure 13.5.

If you continue to apply the Alexander Technique directions accurately, your spine will continue to lengthen in this position (with your spinal curves intact) and you will basically be hinging your whole torso over your hips, knees and ankles. Alexander called this a position of mechanical advantage and worked at helping his students to learn how to get into it reliably. The students in his first teacher training class called it "monkey position."[27] This way of maintaining full stature while lowering your center of gravity and folding your hips and knees and ankles over your base of support provides the basic skills for the more advanced abilities of deeper squatting, as well as lunging and lifting.

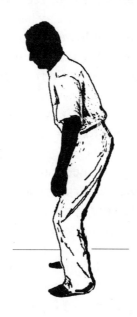

**Figure 13.5 — Folding In Standing:
Squat ("Monkey") Position**

If you're not sure of what you're doing, it's not a scandal to get help. Take your time to clarify the instructions and to observe what you actually do as carefully and accurately as you can.

When you are clear about this basic folding or squatting maneuver, you can begin to apply it to activities like lowering yourself to wash your hands, picking up something from the floor, sitting down, etc. I suggest following Alexander's steps:

1. Start with the idea of lowering yourself at the sink to wash your hands (for example).

2. Pause—inhibit carrying out the action.

3. Give yourself the basic directions, i.e. freeing your neck, to let your head balance up off the end of your spine, to allow your torso to lengthen and widen, etc.

4. Go back to the idea of lowering yourself by folding…at which time you can again pause and direct without carrying out the action …or

5. Continuing to direct yourself to lengthen, let your knees go forwards and out from your hips, hips releasing as you lower your center and bring yourself to the sink.

6. Once you've lowered yourself to the level you need …return to observing your head, neck and back. Have you been able to continue to lengthen, widen and maintain your full stature? [28]

This process may seem unduly drawn out. However, it remains one of the best ways I know to learn how to experience your full stature every day as you fold rather than bend. If you practice in this way, you will learn how to "think in activity" (inhibit and direct) more quickly and more easily as you move. Eventually, moving with awareness can become a habit.

Chapter 14

Design Your Environment

Some of you may remember a famous scene from the 1950s television show "I Love Lucy," in which Lucille Ball's character gets work in a candy factory boxing chocolates on an assembly line. The candy moves faster and faster down the conveyor belt. Lucy stuffs the chocolates everywhere, into the boxes, into her mouth, into her clothing, etc., to no avail. More and more, faster and faster, those 'damned' chocolates keep on coming.

The science of ergonomics studies how to fit the work environment to the worker.[1] All too often, as in Lucy's example, exactly the opposite happens. We end up fitting our selves to our environments, not only at work but also at home and at play.

Our environments include the objects we interact with and their spatial arrangement. They also involve the time element, the rhythm and schedule of activity that comprise our daily life-style.

The third and fourth guidelines for 'mindful' body mechanics will help you take control of your personal ergonomics. They are: *Design your personal environment for better use; Practice postural variety in your daily life*. These two guidelines build on what you already have learned. They also work together and reinforce each other. They are based on the premise that you have some control over your environment and can better shape it to suit yourself.

In this chapter, I present some things to consider when assessing and modifying your personal environment. In the following chapter, I offer some simple steps for increasing postural variety in your daily life. Some of these comments serve as a review of previous material, here specifically applied to guidelines three and four.

Your Personal Environment

Your personal environment, your life space, includes the clothes you wear, external aids like eyeglasses, furniture and placement of furniture at home and work, car seating, etc. What standards do you apply to decide whether your life space helps or hinders your use?

The criteria that I have presented in previous chapters can serve as general guidelines for your efforts to improve your personal environment. Basically, change seems warranted if any aspect of your personal environment reduces the factor-of-safety motion in your joints and keeps you from functioning at your full stature. This includes any environment that encourages monotonous or asymmetrical end range positioning and repetitive forces on your spine and other joints.

As an example of how to explore alternatives, I will briefly discuss a few typical problems and solutions below. Since your problems are unique, what I suggest may not precisely apply to you. You can adapt the suggestions or seek professional advice if you need more intensive problem solving.

Clothing

Let's look at clothing, the part of the environment closest to your skin. Its effect on your body and use may be easy to ignore. Tight jeans, for example, can restrict movement in hips and legs in such a way that folding with a lengthened spine becomes impossible. This means that someone wearing such jeans will be forced to bend with the lower back flexed. Solution?—wear looser-fitting slacks, at least when you're going to squat or lift.

Inadequate or inappropriate shoes also can create literal 'sore points' for body use. Take high heels, for example. A woman wearing high heels is basically standing on her toes. There also is tremendous pressure on her heels. This type of shoe has a strong tendency to push the lower back into an extreme of lordosis, an end range position which, if held without respite, may contribute to strain and pain.

Street and athletic shoes that have gotten worn out or that don't provide adequate pressure relief or support can also contribute to back problems. Simply becoming aware of these difficulties will provide some obvious solutions, i.e., new shoes, a padded insert, etc. A visit to a podiatrist for advice may also help a great deal.

Become aware of the choices you make when you buy clothes and shoes. To what extent do you want fashion to serve as a guide? To what extent do you want freedom of movement to prevail? What other criteria do you use? Answers to these questions can serve as important wedges of awareness.

Vision Aids

Poor vision also can create problems for use. Difficulties with vision often can lead to eyestrain and to protruding your head and neck to get closer to what you are trying to view or read. Larger print for ease of reading, a reading stand, better lighting, a new eyeglass prescription, and vision aids such as a hand magnifier or a screen magnifier for your computer are some of the things that can help you to modify your visual environment. In this way, you can reduce the need to strain and misuse your eyes, head, neck and back.

Seating

Have you taken a good look at your favorite chairs and sofa? Seating that makes it easy for you to sit erect with the full length of your stature may be difficult to come by. Sometimes, as I mentioned previously, a simple dining room or kitchen chair may serve you best. Once you've learned how to sit upright unsupported, you can assess what any particular seat may require to make upright sitting as easy as possible.[2]

In general, as previously mentioned, any seat at least ought to allow your knees to rest squarely at hip joint level. However, having your knees even a bit lower than your hips often can be beneficial as it can makes sitting with some lordosis easier.[3] If the seat height is not adjustable, you can use a small wedge (don't confuse this with the "wedge of awareness") or cushion(s) on the seat to elevate your hips.

Does your seat allow your feet to rest on the floor? If not, perhaps you need a different chair. Lowering the seat if possible or placing supports under your feet, e.g., phone books, may provide another solution.

What about the seat depth, the distance from front edge to chair back? This should give your thighs support without digging into the backs of your knees when you sit against the backrest. If the seat isn't deep enough, you probably need another chair. If it seems too deep, you may be able to place some large cushions or other firm support to fill in some of the extra space behind your back.

What about lumbar support? As mentioned previously, if you have benefited from a lumbar support you may be better off using a portable one that you can move and reposition, rather than one that is built into the chair (unless this is adjustable).

The firmness of the seat bottom and of the chair back are also important factors. Sagging chair backs and bottoms mean that your own back and bottom are likely to sag as well. New upholstery sometimes helps. Sometimes you can modify sagging furniture with extra padding, pillows or supports, even boards. Sometimes, though, you may be better off selling or giving away your chair or sofa.

Alternative types of seating are definitely worth exploring. High stools and perches that allow you to rest midway between standing and the 'normal' sitting position are available. These can make it easier to rest your legs while retaining the normal curves of your spine.

Another alternative is the Scandinavian "Balans" chair that tilts the pelvis forwards while supporting the knees. This also encourages sitting with the natural spinal curves.

People have also experimented using large blow-up gymnastic balls as seats. If your balance is adequate, a ball large enough to sit on with your knees slightly lower than your hips can allow you to sit upright and lengthened while allowing gentle movement.

Beds

Occasionally, some people may feel better sleeping on a sagging surface. However, for the most part, firmer means better, up to a point. Most people do better with pillows and beds that support and encourage the naturally lengthening curves of the spine — not too soft, not too hard, just right.

Sometimes sag occurs, not because of your mattress, but rather because of inadequate mattress support such as worn bedsprings. In this case, placing a plywood board under the mattress sometimes can provide the necessary amount of firmness.

If extending your spine and avoiding flexed postures has helped you, you may need to work on not curling up into a fetal position at night. Although you can't control what happens while you sleep, you can start out in a more neutral position on your back, or on your side with your legs more or less extended and your back lengthened.

You also can support your lumbar curve by sleeping with a lumbar roll. Use a rolled-up bath towel, with a diameter of several inches and held together by rubber bands. Folding the towel in half first can make rolling it a bit easier. If you lay out the belt of a bathrobe inside the towel before you roll it, you can use the protruding ends of the belt to tie the roll around your middle. Commercial devices are also available.[4]

Your pillow provides the sleeping surface for your head and neck. Sleeping with too many pillows can encourage prolonged flexed, protruded or asymmetrically tilted head and neck positions. In general, a thinner pillow can work better than a thicker one to keep your head and neck in alignment with the rest of your spine. Also, in general, I advise people to use a pillow that has some sort of movable stuffing rather than a solid fill. The movable stuffing will conform better to the shape and weight of your head.

If you have had neck problems when lying down, using a neck roll for support often can help. You can use a small towel, rolled up to give it its maximum length. The roll can measure a few inches in diameter—just large enough to support the space under your neck without bringing your head and neck out of neutral alignment as your head rests on the pillow. This can be placed inside the pillowcase along the lower edge of your pillow. A cylinder of foam of similar size can sometimes work well. Commercial neck rolls and pillows are available.[5]

Of course, these are general suggestions. Your particular problems are specific to you. Therefore you may need to make very specific adjustments to suit your distinctive needs. If you have a sore back or neck when lying down at night, you would do well to get individualized advice about sleeping surfaces and positions from a professional as part of a comprehensive evaluation.

Other Home Furnishings

Your home has many surfaces, areas and furnishings that can help or hinder healthful body mechanics to some degree or other. These may include storage cupboards and shelves;

desks, tables and counters to work upon, eat from, etc.; and other furnishings such as toilets, sinks, tubs, showers, etc., to use and to navigate around.

As with many aspects of design, there are standard or average dimensions for these parts of the home environment. Since the average remains that which no one individual quite 'is', this can be a problem.

One factor is paramount — your individuality. We all have the same parts, more or less. But our heights, shapes, sizes, etc., can vary considerably. For example, two people with torsos that are more-or-less the same length may have different arm and leg lengths. With clothing it's somewhat easier to mix and match various sizes and dimensions to suit your individual size and shape than it is with furniture and other parts of your life space.

The dimensions of individual furnishings need to suit you. If you are able to get your home furnishings constructed to suit your personal dimensions you're lucky. Sometimes, for things like counter and sink heights, a readymade variety of dimensions may be available from which to choose. Adjustable height surfaces may be available. If not, it may still be possible to make adjustments.

As a general rule, a work surface should allow you to sit and stand at your full stature without crouching or reaching. That means that you shouldn't have to stay bent over in order to use a work surface.[6] You also should not have to continually reach above shoulder height.

To create an optimal life space, you need to consider the mutual relations of the different parts of your personal environment. How you arrange things within storage areas and upon work surfaces, as well as the spacing and arrangement of your furniture, sometimes can make a tremendous difference for your ease of use. An overly crowded and constricted space may encourage you to constrict yourself. Since your personal environment likely includes others, you will also need to consider the dimensions of those who share your space. How can you negotiate and arrange things in a friendly fashion so that all involved can function at their best?

The criteria that I have presented in previous chapters can help serve as general guidelines for your efforts to improve the surfaces and spaces of your environment:

• To what extent will you need to get into and maintain cramped, awkward, asymmetrical, end range positions?

• Can all of the joints of your body function with some factor–of–safety motion?

• Are you able to work at your full stature, sitting or standing?

• Are things arranged to encourage postural variety? This will be discussed further in the next chapter.

Car Seating

The same advice regarding chairs and other seating applies to car seats. Car seat design has, to some extent, improved over the years. Adjustable built-in lumbar supports can be helpful. Portable wedges, lumbar rolls, etc., can be used to modify even less-than-desirable seating. Consider the seating as part of a new car purchase decision.

At Work

A reasonably humane society will provide a safe and pleasant work environment for all workers. What that actually means in concrete terms for workers in both sedentary and more active occupations seems a matter for some debate.

For more sedentary occupations, desks, chairs, computer keyboards, mice, computer displays, etc., provide multiple opportunities for encouraging misuse. The previous discussion on home seating and work surfaces applies at the office as well.

Some occupations involve tending machinery, frequent lifting, etc., even so-called 'sedentary' office jobs. Evidence exists that frequent, heavy lifting in awkward positions may be encouraged by cramped and otherwise unsuitable work spaces and can cause spinal damage.[7] Vibrating machinery and vehicles, etc., may increase the possibility of injury for workers not protected by vibration-reducing equipment and seating.

We can hope that workers and employers can work together to pinpoint specific hazards and develop reasonable solutions for the work environment. For example, dollies, forklifts and environmental re-design can reduce some of the dangers of repeated heavy lifting, etc. Vibration-dampening springs and seats can be used to protect workers from shaking equipment.

Sometimes environmental design for better body mechanics may require changing job requirements, scheduling and the number of workers employed. For example, nurses and nursing aides have consistently high rates of back injuries.[8] Could this have something to do with their typical work environments? Nursing homes and hospitals often operate with too few caretakers who have too many patients requiring full or partial lifting in the course of their daily care. One or two patients needing such help may put an undue burden on already overworked hospital staff and on the patients for whom they're trying to give good care.

Those hospitals and nursing homes that want to reduce the significant problems with back injuries among the nursing staff have many possible solutions available to improve the work environment. These may include, among other things: extra staffing, flexible staffing, readily available ergonomic aids such as patient lifting devices and other assistive devices for patient care. Note: industrial back belt devices may seem to provide adequate support for preventing back problems. Research suggests otherwise.[9] Don't allow yourself to be fooled.

My own emphasis is on helping people learn and flexibly apply basic principles of use. First and foremost, whatever work situation you find yourself in, realize that it is possible to improve your working environment, sometimes with very simple changes. Persist in your search for a better way! And as you design and reshape your work and other environments to better suit your needs, include the need for postural variety as discussed in the next chapter.

Chapter 15

Increase Your Postural Variety

Children's attention spans drive them to shift and move often during their waking hours. By the time we hit adulthood, however, we have learned to hold our attention to external tasks for longer and longer periods of time. This may mean that we spend longer and longer periods in one or more restricted positions, making limited, repeated and stereotyped movements. We can call this combination of prolonged positioning and/or stereotyped movement *postural monotony*. [Note: I am using the term "postural" here as shorthand for "posture-movement" which I intend to refer to both static and dynamic aspects of your posture-movement habits.]

Postural monotony becomes a problem when it leads you to find it more and more difficult to maintain your full stature easily. When this occurs, you may begin to sag—the protective muscles don't work as well so that spinal joints move into end range and lose their factor-of-safety. As a result, you can feel fatigue and a sense of strain or even pain. After a period of postural monotony, you may feel stiff and 'rickety', when the tissues, which have temporarily adapted to one position, begin to move again.

Postural variety, on the other hand, involves allowing enough change of position and movement throughout the day such that you can keep strain and fatigue to a minimum.[1]

As you develop greater body awareness, you naturally will tend to become more responsive to your own needs for postural variety. You live in a universe of rhythm and change that includes *you*. Can you stand absolutely still with no movement at all? No! You breathe, your heart beats, your blood flows, etc. Just listening more often to your own internal feedback can tell you if change needs to happen. As you're reading this, do you feel any need to shift or stretch? Go ahead, yawn, stretch, move!

Designing Your Environment for Variety

As noted in the previous chapter, promoting postural variety is an important criterion to follow when you look at ways to design your personal environment. As Galen Cranz suggests in her book *The Chair*, "Probably the single most important principle of body-conscious design is to use design to keep posture varied and the body moving."[2] How you arrange things in the space around you can enhance your efforts to vary your posture and thus increase your sense of comfort and your ability to operate efficiently.

For example, you may have an arrangement which allows you to file while still remaining at your desk. However, you may encourage better use by having your file cabinet placed so that you have to stand up from your desk and walk a few steps to file things.

If you have a multi-task job to do, you might consider creating various stations that allow you to do different phases of the work in different places and positions.

If you have alternative types of seating available, you may be able occasionally to switch chairs in your work area during the day. A reading stand may allow you to do some work while standing. Some types of seating, such as a gymnastic ball, will encourage you to move while using them.

The ability to alternate work and rest can also be built into your environment. Do you have a place at home or work where you easily can get into the constructive rest position? The basic idea is to design your environment to allow for greater possibilities for healthful alterations of position and movement. This is somewhat different from the old "time and motion studies" approach to work efficiency, since body awareness has primary importance here.

Relieving Postural Monotony

It's probably inevitable that you will sometimes continue some positions or unidirectional movements longer than you would have liked. In either case, you can follow a simple postural variety principle: *Get out of prolonged positions or repeated directions of movement as soon as possible and go the other way.*[3] This principle can help you reduce strain and prevent pain and irritation to your back and other parts of your body.

The most common monotonous positions and movements for the back involve flexion. Flexion frequently occurs with prolonged sitting and repeated bending. Let's look at how to apply the postural variety principle to these common activities.

You can learn how to sit with better body mechanics for longer periods of time. However, despite your best intentions, the best seating, lumbar supports, etc., if you sit long enough you will tend to start losing your full stature and go into some degree of flexion.

Therefore, when sitting gets prolonged, follow the corrective principle by getting out of the chair, standing upright and bending backwards (the Extension in Standing exercise in Chapter 10). If you get up frequently enough (before you begin having pain) and bend backwards five or six times, you will be doing yourself a tremendous favor. You may feel some stiffness at first. This should ease up with repetitions of the backward-bending movement. If you notice increasing or peripheralizing pain or other symptoms as you repeat the movement, stop. You may need to get professional advice.

Slumped sitting can also involve protruding your head and neck in front of your spine and torso. A corrective to the protruded head and neck position is to …that's right… *move them the other way* with the chin-tuck exercise (head/neck retraction).[4] This has also been called the "hen" exercise because the movement of your head back and forth looks something like the movements a hen makes when it walks.[5]

This movement, used by many rehabilitation professionals, goes in the opposite direction of the protruded head position. Remember that with the protruded position you poke your head and neck in front of the rest of your body. At the extreme of this position, your head will be tilted backwards in relation to your upper neck while your lower cervical area will be flexed more (making the upper back "hump" you've quite likely seen).

To do the chin-tuck movement, sit or stand upright. Now move your head and neck back over the rest of your spine. If your eyes continue to look forwards, you will be bringing your chin in (tucking it) closer to your throat, while your head actually tilts forwards and moves up in relation to your upper neck. The flexed hump in your lower neck area will reduce.

Go as far as you can in this direction (you can add a little guidance and extra stretch with one or two hands on your chin gently pushing backwards). Return to a relaxed position (no need to return to an exaggeratedly protruded one) and then repeat the tuck motion five to ten times. Figure 15.1 illustrates the movement.

As with the lower back exercise, you may feel strain initially with this movement but this should not increase as you repeat it. If you feel increasing or peripheralizing pains or other symptoms, don't persist. These corrective movements can be done whenever you have been sitting for a prolonged period, as, for example, with long car rides, plane trips, sitting in a meeting, a classroom or in a theatre. Whenever you can do so, take a break, get out of your seat, stand and move the other way. When you find it difficult to get out of your seat, you may still be able to move your spine to some degree in the opposite direction.

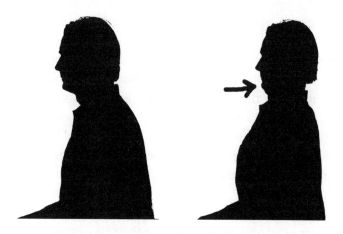

Figure 15.1 – Hen Exercise (Chin-Tuck)

Repeated or prolonged bending activities in standing might include such activities as vacuuming, shoveling, gardening and lifting. The elegant solution regarding these activities involves doing them with your full stature in a biomechanically advantageous manner. In other words, you will do these activities by folding in a way that keeps your spine in a lengthened state. However, some of us may fall short of this at least some of the time. Even when you use yourself well, these activities may cause strain if repeated or prolonged enough. Therefore, you need to get out of this kind of position with some frequency and…that's right…*go the other way*. Five to ten standing backbends at sufficient intervals during an activity may be enough to avoid the onset of problems.

Postural Variety and Fitness

At one time, most people didn't have to worry about getting enough exercise. Vigorous physical activity was the rule for a much larger percentage of the population. For example, if people wanted to get somewhere, for the most part they walked. Of course, life wasn't perfect and more people may have suffered from 'back-breaking' physical labor than at present.

Now, sedentary occupations are much more common. Many people spend most, if not all, of their working hours sitting. Many of us may consider ourselves lucky in not having to work very hard doing physical labor in order to survive. Yet this has led in part to other problems, such as what some observers see as a rise in 'back-breaking' *inactivity*, as well as obesity and stress-related disorders. Both for your back and for your general well-being, find/create more posture-movement variety for yourself by increasing your activity and fitness level.

You can start by making an honest account of your daily activities for a week. What percentage of the time do you sit, walk, stand, lie down (rest), sleep (in what position?), exercise (doing what?), sports and recreation (what and how much?) in a typical day?... in a typical week? Analyze the data you've collected. Is there some type of activity that you don't get enough of? It doesn't seem as if most people have the problem of not sitting enough.

If you get little or no physical exercise, you can start to get more, here and now. If you are over the age of 35 or have a current medical condition, including pain or other symptoms, consult your medical doctor first.[6]

Aerobic activities (those that improve cardiovascular conditioning) provide a good basis for any exercise program. Walking remains among the simplest and easiest of aerobic activities. Done for 30 to 40 minutes, 3 to 4 times per week at a level of comfortable exertion, a walking program can provide a good foundation for a general exercise program.[7]

It is better to start slowly and easily. Don't push too hard. Rather, do less that you think you can do. You can start by walking one block for example, then gradually progress to two blocks, three blocks, half a mile, a mile, etc. As you walk, take a few wedges of awareness to free your neck, let your head balance forwards and up on top of your lengthening spine, to let your back and torso lengthen and widen.

You will need to decide for yourself how much exercise is enough for you. No absolute rule exists. Reporting on exercise research, Washington Post writer Carol Krucoff states, "Lifestyle activity—such as taking the stairs instead of the elevator and parking in the farthest space rather than the one closest to your destination—can provide health benefits similar to those of a traditional, gym-based workout, according to a 1997 study called Project Active, performed at the Cooper Institute for Aerobics Research in Dallas." [8] There are a number of components that enter into "physical fitness," including cardiovascular endurance, flexibility, strength, coordination, balance, etc. Different programs of exercise may emphasize these components in varying degrees and in different ways. Your choices about what and how much to do will be influenced by your health needs and your recreational interests.

If you have started a basic walking program and are looking for more vigorous workouts, you can explore aerobics exercises such as running, or group classes such as aerobic dance, kickboxing, etc. Strength training may be useful as well and has been shown to help people recovering from back injuries and those who have been dealing with chronic pain. To avoid unnecessary problems make sure you have a qualified instructor and have necessary medical clearance. Find out about any special classes for people who have had back problems. Those that feature "spinal stabilization" may have particular usefulness.

Your back health and safety must be a major consideration in any exercise program you do in addition to a basic walking program. My personal favorite as an exercise system is the gentle, awareness-based approach of Tai Chi. I have practiced this graceful movement discipline since 1985. Tai Chi began in China as a martial art, yet can be done purely for exercise. It can help you to develop greater balance and coordination. The principles and practice of Tai Chi reinforce the body mechanics approach of the Alexander Technique. Tai Chi is related to a whole group of exercises called Qigong, which you also may find useful to explore.

You can find Tai Chi instructors in more and more places. Observe a class or two, talk with the instructor, find out about the person's philosophy and background, and choose one who seems right for you. Forms of practice may vary but teachers of whatever type follow a central core of posture and movement-related principles. I advise choosing a teacher who can help you learn the practical aspects that can be done without the need to follow any belief system.[9]

Yoga can also provide a 'mindful' approach to exercise. There are many different forms, some more vigorous than others. Flexibility and breathing receive special emphasis. Again, find an experienced teacher who emphasizes practical aspects and can individualize the instruction to fit your particular needs.

It can be useful to discuss your individual health concerns with an appropriate health-care provider. Your personal physician will be able to give you general guidelines on exercise related to your back and other health issues you may have. A physician may also be able to provide you with advice about how to get more information on exercise to meet your personal health and life-style goals. A rehabilitation professional, such as a physical therapist, can also advise you on exercise issues related to any activity-related back or other movement problems you have had.

For questions related to recreational sports, you might do well to get additional advice from a professional instructor in that particular activity. For example, if you like to ski you can get advice from a professional ski instructor on the kind of conditioning that you need to ski safely at your skill level and to get to the next level as well.

Whatever exercises and sports you do, remember the importance of *how* you do what you do, *your use*. Robert Rickover, Alexander Technique teacher and author of the book *Fitness Without Stress*, has written that "It isn't only the number of miles run, the time spent doing aerobic exercises, or the heaviness of the weights lifted that matters. Far more important is the *quality* of our movements — our balance and coordination and our ease of breathing."[10] An Alexander Technique teacher can help you learn to apply the principles of good use and body mechanics to improve the quality of any of your fitness activities. Applying the principles of good use to your other activities of daily living will enable you to enjoy what I call "the athleticism of everyday life" as well.

Postural Variety and Rest

Perhaps we could call this the Age of Faster But Not Necessarily Better. With all the 'labor-saving' and 'time-saving' devices we have, such as cellular phones, pagers and faster, more powerful computers and internet connections, many people have more work with less time to do it.

This makes it even more important to include rest as a necessary element in finding/creating posture-movement variety for yourself. Look again at your daily and weekly account of activities. How much time do you allow for sleep? How much time for resting during the day? As devotees of 'faster', many of us don't give ourselves sufficient time for sleep or for adequate rest.

This can have a significant effect on back and other musculoskeletal problems. With fatigue, we can easily become more preoccupied and inattentive to what we are doing. Judgment may get reduced. We can sag into our joints more easily, moving out of our factor–of–safety range and into stress-ful, sustained end range positions. The protective functions of the muscles may not work as quickly to protect our joints from sudden stresses and jolts.

One of the minimum pieces of 'homework' I ask clients to do is to lie down for 15 to 20 minutes at least once a day in constructive rest position. I often have to persist in this request from week to week because, as easy as it seems, many people don't find it easy to get themselves to do it even once a day.

Rest is not an absolute but a relative quality. One of the 'secrets' of efficient movement mechanics is what writer Aldous Huxley called "relaxation in activity."[11] This quality of rest and repose during skilled activity can be seen clearly in performances of great skill such as the play of Tiger Woods and Michael Jordan, the dancing of Ginger Rogers and Fred Astaire, and the piano technique of Artur Rubinstein. Anato-mist and anthropologist Raymond Dart, M.D., a student of the Alexander Technique and of human movement, said, "In ev-ery game and craft perfect relaxation of the unwanted muscles is the key to skilled performance."[12]

A simple way to begin experiencing more of this sense of relaxation in activity is to practice pausing when you can in the midst of an activity. Give yourself a wedge of awareness and ask yourself a few questions suggested by Milton Trager, M.D., founder of the Trager approach to movement education: *What can feel freer? What can feel easier? What can feel lighter?*[13]

Find out what needs less tension, more movement, and experience your sense of your body there. For example, per-haps you have been sitting at the computer for awhile. Your hand has been pressing onto the mouse and feels tight and tense. Let go and let your arm hang at your side. Give your hand a gentle shake so that you can feel your thumb and each of your fingers move. How can you let this movement feel easier, softer, lighter? Allow the movement to go into your wrist, forearm, elbow, arm, shoulder. After about a minute let your hand rest. Notice any changes. Does this hand feel any different from the other one? As you bring your hand back to the mouse, how can you continue feeling lighter and easier there? Practicing this kind of gentle, 'mindful' movement can help you to avoid undue effort and find more relaxation in more of what you do.

A related principle of use is one elaborated by John Mennell, M.D., that I call *relative rest*.[14] When recovering from an injury, you may not need to stop moving the injured part completely. Rather, you can find a certain threshold of activity, which, if you stay below it, will allow you to be active to some degree without impairing the healing process. Indeed, relative activity during relative rest can help you feel and function better sooner.

Sometimes easing up on one particular kind of activity, position or movement may be sufficient. In addition, as you recover from injury you may be able to begin regular activities just by reducing the speed or duration of a particular movement.[15] This is useful to remember in athletics and also when you are getting back to doing regular household or work activities. It won't hurt — and will help — to tell yourself to "take it easy," "take it slow" and "take it a little bit at a time," especially if you actually listen to yourself.

You can also use this advice for preventing injuries when starting a new activity or skill. For example, a runner may do well to reduce speed a bit when first adding mileage. In any task that you do, you might do well at first to make haste slowly.

Consult your health care provider as to what activities, positions, etc., to avoid altogether, and for how long. This is especially important when you currently are dealing with back pain. However, staying flat on your back in bed usually is not a useful approach to functioning better faster.

Another contributor to an understanding of rest in daily life is Ernest Rossi, Ph.D., a psychologist who has explored *ultradian rhythms*. These are daily biological rhythms that occur during our period of waking consciousness. Ultradian rhythms involve times of externalized, focused activity of around 90 minutes in length, interspersed with more internalized periods of brain/body restoration and repose of around 20 minutes in length.

Be assured that when you find yourself daydreaming, going to the water cooler, looking for a snack, or yawning or stretching during your workday, you are doing what comes naturally. These ultradian periods of rest do not necessarily come at the time that your boss schedules a coffee break. They come as part of a natural cycle and are related to body posture and use. You can learn to make use of these times more consciously.

By recognizing when you seem to be entering a "rest" period, for example if you are having difficulty concentrating, you can learn how to make the most of it rather than fight it. If it is possible, this can be a good time to stretch, yawn, get up and move around, get a snack or take a nap.

If you can do it, a twenty-minute nap can be just the thing you need to restore yourself for the next phase of working activity. Winston Churchill, a great leader against Nazi tyranny during World War II, was known for his ability to take a quick nap, sometimes for just a few minutes, when he had the opportunity. Churchill helped save the free world and I guess the naps didn't hurt.

Employers often short-sightedly think that their workers need to be 'busy' and buzzing around like worker bees the entire day in order to function efficiently. This unphysiological 'nonsense' may lead to exactly the opposite result. More is not necessarily better. In a more enlightened time, perhaps we can expect employers to provide more opportunities for their employees to nap openly. It remains to be seen what effects this could have on rates of back injuries.

If a nap doesn't seem practical, just pausing to look out of a window, take a deep breath or close your eyes for a moment will help you to function better. If you're feeling tired or distracted, changing how you sit, looking into the distance, moving into a new position or shifting to a new activity also can help to revive you. Different tasks may require different amounts of attention. Moving to a routine and relatively 'mindless' task may be useful after work requiring a high degree of concentration.

You can pump up your ability to stay awake and alert by taking breaks, taking a nap, ingesting caffeine, exercising, etc. This only goes so far. You can't stay awake and alert forever. Eventually, getting adequate rest means that you must get sufficient sleep.

Inadequate sleep will lead to excessive fatigue which will interfere with your ability to function and feel better with less pain. If the demands from work and home become extreme, you may neglect or feel unable to sleep sufficiently. In addition, pain may interfere with your ability to sleep well and thus may contribute to a spiral of more fatigue and pain.

Discuss any sleep problems you have with your medical doctor.[16] If pain interferes with your sleep, the proper medications can help. Getting help in dealing with emotional stresses also can make a difference. Take care of other underlying medical problems, such as allergies, that may interfere with sleep. Sleep disorders are gaining greater recognition and more physicians specializing in this area are available if specialized testing or treatment seems needed.

Guidelines for Reducing Stress

Stress expert Hans Selye, M.D., once said "Variety of experience is not only the spice of life but possibly the key to longer life."[17] Practicing postural variety may not increase your life span but, along with the other rules of 'mindful' body mechanics, it can help you live the life you have with greater ease and effectiveness.

Here again are the four general rules of 'mindful' use:

1. *Make body awareness a daily practice.*

2. *Experience your full stature everyday as often as you can.*

3. *Design your personal environment for better use.*

4. *Practice postural variety in your daily life.*

As the last four chapters show, these flexible guidelines work together. By finding small ways to apply these principles in your everyday life, you can use them to develop better posture-movement habits for yourself. To the extent that the pain you've experienced depends on your use, these principles can help you reduce your musculoskeletal stress and gain greater control of your life.

Conclusion

The obscure we see eventually;
the completely apparent takes longer.
- Edward R. Murrow[1]

Chapter 16

Preventing Back Pain

Problems and Solutions

Back pain problems have vexed humans throughout history. Documented records of back pain and sciatica go as far back as the ancient Egyptians and Greeks.[1] Starting in the latter half of the twentieth century, there has occurred a documented rise in healthcare expenses and in lost productivity due to back pain disability. Does this indicate a significant change in the percentage of the population experiencing back pain now as compared with previous times? Not necessarily. Some have suggested that the rise in disability related to back pain may have come about more as an unintended consequence of some of the measures (such as inappropriate illness benefits) used to deal with the problem.[2] Some so-called solutions—passive treatments and rest—may have resulted not only in increased disability but in diagnostic confusions and treatment impasses as well.

However, the situation is changing. Many health care professionals now recognize that common back pain has important mechanical (activity-related or, as I have termed it, posture-movement-related) aspects. Treatments now put a greater emphasis on the use of activity and exercise. There is also greater recognition of the need to understand the biopsychosocial nature of back pain—how mechanical and other so-called physical factors interact with a person's psychological states and social environments.

Unfortunately, these understandings may get little more than lip service. Practitioners may not go beyond giving generalized advice on attitude, activity and exercise. If each person with back pain functions as a unique individual, such general advice is not sufficient. A broadly interpreted scientific attitude sees the individual as paramount. Therefore, treatments and advice need to be tailored specifically to each individual's condition.

The posture-movement model of pain and recovery (presented in Chapter 9) provides a biopsychosocial framework for understanding your individual condition. The therapy and education guidelines which follow this will help you to function as a personal scientist in relation to your individual back problem. Using the guidelines for posture-movement therapy (presented in Chapter 10) you can explore how different, specific positions and movements may produce, increase, decrease or abolish your symptoms. Applying the guidelines for posture-movement education (presented in Part IV) you can explore how your particular moment-to-moment posture-movement habits (your body mechanics/use) affect how you function. Can applying these principles help you as an individual to deal more effectively with back pain? I think so.

Personal and Group Research

There is a great deal that we don't know about back pain. More definitive answers to many questions will require a great deal more high quality research than has presently been done. Such research will include using statistical studies of large groups of people in randomized, controlled clinical trials. This kind of research is difficult to do well, can be misinterpreted and may neglect or downplay the factor of individuality. Nonetheless, such studies are needed to make good generalizations about the percentage (relative frequency) of people in similar groupings who can be presumed to respond (or not respond) to various treatments.

However, it seems like a great mistake to assume that no other kinds of data have value or that we don't know anything now. Dr. Stephen Barrett and Dr. William Jarvis, two advocates for high quality information and research in healthcare, have pointed out that, "Although controlled trials are important, many scientific truths are derived from other types of careful observation."[3]

Many different types of evidence point to the value of the principles of posture-movement therapy and education. I have provided references for some of this evidence in the Notes section. I include as evidence the kinds of observations you can make in your own personal research to explore your possibilities for feeling better. You don't need to take my word for it or accept questionable beliefs or practices. With very little expense, you—as a personal scientist—can test, in your own life-laboratory, the power of posture-movement principles, using this book as your lab manual.

Admittedly, there are limitations to this kind of personal research. Individuals can easily jump to definite conclusions about cause and effect relations between treatments and results, based on their fallible and limited experience. It is easy for individuals to fool themselves and/or be fooled by others. That's how quackery works. In the case of back pain, we can mistakenly confuse the presumed benefits of a given treatment with the actual benefits of the passage of time alone. In actuality, reasonable conclusions about health matters are often difficult to reach. Nonetheless, an advantage of a posture-movement approach is that it is sometimes very easy to observe immediate cause and effect relations among positions, movements and signs/symptoms.

Another related limitation of the kind of personal research discussed above is the difficulty in making very definitive conclusions about groups of people based on the experience of one or a few persons. This doesn't mean that anecdotal evidence should simply be tossed aside. Rather, conclusions suggested by anecdotal or case evidence need to be held rather tentatively until supported by further research that allows greater generalization.

I have used and documented the benefits of posture-movement therapy and education for my individual clients, as have many other therapists who use such methods. I may be wrong, but my experience strongly suggests that for most people, the kind of posture-movement therapy I discuss in this book, in combination with posture-movement education such as the Alexander Technique, is superior to other methods presently used for common back problems.

I'd like to highlight here two studies which support this view. One focused on chronic pain patients; they were found to experience significant improvements in pain relief and the ability to function when using the McKenzie Method of posture-movement therapy.[4] In another study, the Alexander Technique was taught as part of a comprehensive pain management approach for chronic pain patients. Patients rated these posture-movement education sessions as one of the most significant interventions they experienced.[5]

These studies suggest great possibilities, but more detailed and comprehensive long term studies with controls need to be done. What outcomes might result from a well-designed program for back patients that integrates posture-movement therapy, for example the McKenzie approach, with posture-movement education using the Alexander Technique? I predict greater benefits compared with other kinds of treatment. Controlled studies done with large groups of people testing this hypothesis have yet to be done. In the meantime smaller, less extensive research studies continue to show the promise of posture-movement therapy and education.

Preventing Back Pain

Is it possible to prevent back pain using the principles of this book? I think so. But I can't say with the utmost certainty. Unfortunately, we so far lack the strongest level of scientific evidence here. Large scale, controlled studies will need to be carried out in order to more definitely determine whether it is possible to reduce the number of episodes of back pain in the general population, reduce the duration of episodes, reduce the severity and frequency of recurrences, and reduce the time away from normal activities and work. However, I believe that some preliminary evidence exists and that the question is worth pursuing.

I have had a number of episodes of neck and back pain over my adult years. As I have learned and applied the principles in this book, I have been able to reduce the severity, duration and frequency of these episodes. Although I have modified my activities at times, I have never had to take time off from work for back or neck pain. My posture, as noted by a number of independent observers, has improved as I have gotten older.

I have observed and recorded similar results with the clients who have come to me with back and neck problems. Other practitioners using the kinds of posture-movement therapy and education described in this book have had similar results. Many different types of published research are available which point to the value of these approaches. Although some may disagree, I believe that at this point enough evidence exists to make it irresponsible of me *not* to present this information here.

One claim that I feel confident in making is that there exists a clear relation between posture (posture-movement habits) and pain. A large body of research supports this. In one study, especially worthy of note, researcher Stover Snook, Ph.D., and colleagues, "showed significant reductions in pain intensity" in individuals with chronic, nonspecific back pain who were taught to control (avoid) lumbar flexion in the early morning hours after waking. Individuals received instructions in how to get out of bed without bending and how to avoid all bending, sitting and squatting for the first two hours (reaching devices were supplied as well as special urinals for the women to use while standing). Participants were instructed that slight bending was okay after two hours and that after six hours they could do their normal activities. Extreme bending was to be avoided at all times.

Participants were required to keep a daily diary to monitor pain intensity, functional disability/impairment and medication use. The control group was given 'sham' exercises to do (these included the traditional pelvic tilts and knees-to-chest exercises favored by flexion enthusiasts). After six months of treatment, participants experienced significant reductions in pain levels (18–29%) compared to the control group (6–9%) and had related reductions in disability/impairment and medication usage. The control group then received the experimental treatment and experienced similar improvements.

The researchers concluded:

In a small sample of relatively unselected subjects with less than 50% compliance, chronic low back pain was significantly reduced without medication, manipulation, exercises, injections, or surgery. The reduction in pain was accomplished by a change in behavior. It was concluded that controlling lumbar flexion in the early morning is a form of self-care that has the potential for reducing pain as well as costs associated with chronic, non-specific low back pain.[6]

Snook's study supports the emphasis in this book on the importance of posture-movement habits as well as the importance of neutral postures, the natural curves of the spine, and reducing the frequency of flexion.

Robert Pula has noted that, "If something goes without saying, it often goes even better *with* saying." It 'goes without saying,' then, that 'bad' posture will not automatically and absolutely guarantee that you *will* have back pain. Rather, it will increase the probability that you may have back pain. Conversely, 'good' posture will not automatically and absolutely guarantee that you will never have back pain. Rather, it will increase the probability that you will have fewer, less severe back problems.

266   **BACK PAIN SOLUTIONS**

Future Directions

I feel fairly sure that, as a society, we will not make significant inroads into preventing back and other musculoskeletal problems until we tackle a number of related issues.

First, *healthcare consumers need to take more responsibility for their own musculoskeletal health. In turn, healthcare providers need to be able to teach them how to do this.* Too many people still look for the magic of passive treatments which too many healthcare providers have been too willing to supply. If you have read this far, I hope that you have begun to realize that the primary responsibilty for your back belongs to you.

As a healthcare consumer you will do well to expect the following from providers:

    • Adequate diagnosis which includes detailed attention to posture-movement factors

    • Individualized instruction in self-treatment using your own positions and movements (exemplified by the McKenzie Method)

    • Manipulative therapy when needed to assist the self-care process and not as a cure-all[7]

    • Adequate individualized instruction in body mechanics based on scientifically-based principles of good use and human learning (exemplified by the Alexander Technique).

Second, *consumers need to look for "body-conscious design" in furniture, automobiles, and living/working environments.* People interested in promoting their musculoskeletal well-being will need to take greater responsibility in designing their own environments. By seeking out seating and equipment that promote better use and postural variety, they will make it more likely that designers, furniture makers, and others will take these issues more seriously.

Third, although the question of workplace ergonomics remains controversial, *businesses need to cooperate with their employees to provide more worker-friendly, 'body'-friendly environments*. Enlightened businesses will work to create pilot projects that can show the effectiveness of ergonomics/alternative management programs to reduce worker injuries and disability expenses. In the long run, this will benefit workers, businesses and society.[8] An important point here: in the workplace as elsewhere, 'psychosocial' and 'physical' factors do not exist as separate elements in isolation from one another. Some occupational health researchers at present seem to believe that they can separate them. In actuality they can only do so verbally.

Fourth, *a concerted effort needs to be made to teach all children the principles of posture-movement care as presented in this book and elsewhere*. Primary prevention of back pain will not happen if children are never encouraged to discover the optimal ways to sit, stand, bend, lift, etc. Elite team sports for the few need to be deemphasized to the extent that they reduce physical education opportunities for all children. Posture-movement education, one of the "non-verbal humanities" (as Aldous Huxley called it)[9], can be integrated with health, music, science and other aspects of the curriculum.

Pilot programs and some initial research have already been done, including the Chelsea, Massachusetts School Survey in 1923-24 where children were taught remedial body mechanics[10], various schools run by F.M. Alexander and/or his students, Ann Mathews' research teaching the Alexander Technique in a public school classroom, Jack Fenton's Alexander Technique–based movement classes with English school children, and Michelle Arsenault's two-year pilot project teaching Alexander Technique-based body mechanics to New York City school children in the context of the science curriculum.

Arsenault's project and her book, *Moving To Learn*, has inspired the founding of The Moving To Learn Society. The Society has the following purposes:

1.   To promote among parents, teachers, school authorities, and the general public the understanding and practice of scientific body mechanics by the school children of this nation, in the interest of both more effective learning and lifelong health and well-being.

2.   To conduct educational activities, including but not limited to conferences, lectures, courses, workshops, publications, and research, relative to the foregoing.[11]

If not taught properly, body mechanics education could become as dull and deadly as the boring sex education class in a Monty Python skit. When taught well the subject of body mechanics and use has a great deal of intrinsic interest for both children and adults. Arsenault's book contains reports from her pilot project and detailed lesson plans that will be of interest to anyone concerned with this subject. Her work teaching children about their own bodies and selves demonstrates the importance not only of the actual content but also of the support and encouragement given them to explore their own capacities.

Fifth, at the other end of the age spectrum, *we need to change our attitudes about older people. Pain and deformity are not inevitable as we grow older.* It is possible to reduce back pain and other types of musculoskeletal pain among the elderly. It is possible, as well, to prevent or reduce the bent, stooped postures that many people associate with old age. I have known many older people, some but not all of them Alexander Technique teachers, who have been able to retain an appearance of poise that younger people might envy. It is best to start young. However, posture-movement habits can be cultivated and improved at any age and surprising changes may occur.

Back to the Source

There is a common source for solutions—not only for back pain, but also for other problems that beset us humans. That common source consists of the natural, childlike potential for learning and change that all of us are born with but gradually tend to lose as we grow older.

We have a great deal to learn from children. In his book *Growing Young*, Ashley Montagu lists some of the valuable traits of childlike (not child*ish*) behavior: curiosity, imaginativeness, playfulness, open-mindedness, willingness to experiment, flexibility, humor, energy, receptiveness to new ideas, honesty, eagerness to learn and the ability to love.[12] It is possible to encourage these qualities in our children and to cultivate and renew them in ourselves.

In this way, you can continue to *grow young* as you age chronologically. If you accept the unity and inseparability of 'mind' and 'body', then these childlike qualities all have a psycho-physical nature.[13] What is the relation of these qualities or their lack to so-called 'physical' and 'mental' health? How do they find expression in your posture-movement patterns?[14] This qualifies as a whole new domain for research that has barely begun to be developed.[15]

In the meantime, you don't need to wait for more formal research or for other people to change. What can you do for yourself right here and now, as you explore your own possibilities for back pain solutions?

Notes

Epigraph

1. Rosten, *Leo Rosten's Treasury of Jewish Quotations*, p. 259

Dedication

1. Yiddish term "rhymes with 'bench.' from German: *Mensch*: 'person.' Plural: *menshen*. 1. A human being...2. An upright, honorable, decent person...3. Someone of consequence; someone to admire and emulate; someone of noble character...To be a *mensh* has nothing to do with success, wealth, status [or gender]. A judge can be a *zhlob*; a millionaire can be a *momzer*; a professor can be a *shlemiel*; a doctor a *klutz*; a lawyer a *bulvon*. The key to being a 'real *mensh*' is nothing less than—character: rectitude, dignity, a sense of what is right, responsible, decorous. Many a poor man, many an ignorant man, is a *mensh*." (Leo Rosten, *The Joys of Yiddish*, p. 237)

Usage Note

1. Qtd. in Kodish and Kodish, pp. 180-181

Introduction

1. Whyte, *The Next Development In Man*, p. 9

Chapter 1

1. Waddell, p.135

2. Waddell, p. 135-136

3. Deyo, p. 50

4. McKenzie's texts for clinicians are *The Lumbar Spine: Mechanical Diagnosis and Therapy*, *The Cervical and Thoracic Spine: Mechanical Diagnosis and Therapy* and *The Human Extremities: Mechanical Diagnosis and Therapy*. McKenzie's more popularly-oriented books are *Treat Your Own Back*, *Treat Your Own Neck* and *7 Steps to a Pain-Free Life*. The application of this approach to other musculoskeletal problems can also be found in Mark Laslett's clinical textbook, *Mechanical Diagnosis and Therapy: The Upper Limb*. McKenzie's work is built upon the pioneering work of Dr. James Cyriax. See Cyriax's *Textbook of Orthopaedic Medicine* and *Illustrated Manual of Orthopaedic Medicine*. The article "Spinal Therapeutics Based On Responses To Loading" by Gary Jacob, D.C., and Robin McKenzie, provides an illuminating and comprehensive presentation of "the underly-

ing philosophic and practical perspectives of the McKenzie approach..." (p.225). See also the articles by John Barbis and by Wayne Rath and Jean Duffy Rath.

5. The term "Cognitive-Kinesthetic Education" comes from Ron Dennis, Ed.D. (personal communication). Michael J. Gelb's book, *Body Learning: An Introduction to the Alexander Technique* and Robert M. Rickover's *Fitness Without Stress* serve as brief introductions for the general reader. Wilfred Barlow, M.D., a physician who studied, taught and did research on the AT, also wrote a sound, science-based and readable introduction, *The Alexander Technique: How To Use Your Body Without Stress*. The essays of *Curiosity Recaptured*, edited by Jerry Sontag, show AT applications to a variety of areas of interest. I also recommend Deborah Caplan's book, *Back Trouble*. Caplan, a physical therapist and Alexander Technique teacher, provided a view that complements my own. F. M. Alexander's own writings are well-worth reading and provide many 'gems' for the serious student. See his *Articles and Lectures: Articles, Published Letters and Lectures on the F. M. Alexander Technique*, edited by Jean M. O. Fischer. Also see *The Books of F. Matthias Alexander* published by IRDEAT (the Institute for Research, Development and Education in the Alexander Technique).

6. Dennis's definition of AT is in his outcome research article on AT and balance, "Functional Reach Improvement in Normal Women After Alexander Technique Instructions."

7. Barrett Dorko's book *Shallow Dive: Essays on the Craft of Manual Care* and the essays on his website (http:barrettdorko.com/index.htm) provide an especially important scientific and humanistic perspective on the effectiveness of such educational methods. Dorko, an innovative and skillful practitioner of physical therapy, has developed *Simple Contact*, a profound way of encouraging pain-relieving activity which involves "...a technique of communication, either verbal or manual, designed to enhance another's awareness and expression of their spontaneously occurring internal processes."

8. "Might not the individual man, each in his own personal way, assume more of the stature of a scientist, ever seeking to predict and control the course of events with which he is involved?" (George A. Kelly, *A Theory of Personality: The Psychology of Personal Constructs*, p. 5)

9. If you have more curiosity about what taking a scientific approach to living entails, read *Drive Yourself Sane: Using the Uncommon Sense of General Semantics*, written by me and my wife, Susan Presby Kodish. Also see the book edited by Susan, *Developing Sanity in Human Affairs*.

10. Howe and Greenburg, p. 496

11. Rosten, p. 302

12. Runkel, pp. 175-176

Part I – Problems and Solutions

1. Allen, quoted by Laurence J. Peter, *Peter's People*, p. 184

Chapter 2

1.This and other stories about patients are as true as I can make them while changing names and other identifying data.

2. Deyo, p. 50

3. Deyo, p. 49

4. See article "Prevalence of Back Pain — By Quality of Study" which reports these figures from the study by R.C. Lawrence et al., "Estimates of the Prevalence of Arthritis and Selected Musculoskeletal Disorders in the United States."

5. Deyo, p. 50

6. Deyo, p. 50-51

7. See Dana Greene's "Abstracts That Discourage Treatment Based on Imaging Results Alone."

8. Boden

9. See Deyo, p. 50 and the article by Cherkin et al., "Physician Variation In Diagnostic Testing For Low Back Pain."

10. Waddell, p. 244

11. Waddell, p. 243

12. See "Major Sciatica Treatment Proves Ineffective In Landmark Randomized Trial," reported in *The Back Letter.* Also see Deyo, pp. 51-52, as well as Bigos, et al., and the Royal College Guidelines.

13. See Bigos et al., under the subheading "Physical Agents and Modalities."

14. Waddell, p. 398

15. McKenzie, *The Lumbar Spine*, p. 2

16. Deyo, p. 51

17. See J.A. Rizzo et al., "The Labor Productivity Effects of Chronic Backache in the United States."

18. See Elaine Thomas et al., "Predicting Who Develops Chronic Low Back Pain in Primary Care: A Prospective Study." "About 30% of patients [in a group of 180 patients studied] continued to have disabling back pain after 12 months."

19. This study was reported on in "Acute Back Pain Benign But Frequently Persistent" in *The Back Letter*. Only 37% of patients studied reported complete pain relief in the study done by Reis and associates printed in "A New Look at Low Back Complaints in Primary Care" in *Journal of Family Practice*, 48 (4): 299-303 (1990) .

20. One study showed disabling recurrences at rates between 8% and 14% from 3 to 6 months after an initial episode. Recurrence rates were 20% to 35% between 6 to 22 months after an initial injury (see Timothy S. Cary, "Recurrence and Care Seeking After Acute Back Pain: Results of a Long-term Follow-up Study").

21. See Deyo, p. 52. Also see Samanta and Beardsley's article, "Low Back Pain: Which is the Best Way Forward?" and "Exercise Beneficial for Low Back Pain" in *PT Bulletin*, August 30, 1999.

22. See Deyo, p. 52.

23. Qtd. in "New UK Back Pain Guidelines" in *The Back Letter*

24. See The American Academy of Orthopaedic Surgeons, *Low Back Pain*, available at www.aaos.org under patient education: spine: patient education brochures.

25. See Moffat and Vickery, pp. 123-124.

26. See the American Chiropractic Association (ACA) "Policies On Public Health."

Chapter 3

1. Licht, in Basmajian, p. 1

2. Cyriax, *Textbook of Orthopaedic Medicine, Vol.1*, p. 484

3. Kamenetz, in Rogoff, p. 8

4. Licht, p. 4

5. Ackerknecht, p. 58

6. Waddell, p. 241

7. Cyriax, op. cit., p. 348

8. Maitland, *Vertebral Manipulation*, p. 3

9. Jacob and McKenzie, p. 225

10. McKenzie, *The Cervical and Thoracic Spine*, p. 103

Chapter 4

1. Waddington, p. 24

2. "What I Believe," in *Alfred Korzybski Collected Writings 1920-1950*, pp. 643-663

3. *Science and Sanity, 5th Edition*, p. liii

4. See Note 1, Chapter 3 above.

5. "Late nineteenth century singing teachers advised students to develop upright posture..., full chest breathing..., and the correct opening of the mouth without any muscular strain..., before the actual singing lessons would start." Staring, p. 135

6. Staring, pp. 205-239

7. Cohen, pp. 27-28

8. Staring, pp. 34-37

9. Licht, pp. 20-23

10. Qtd. by Staring, p. 35

11. In *The Books of F. Matthias Alexander.* New York: IRDEAT

12. Staring's two volume work, *The First 43 Years of the Life of F. M. Alexander*, provides overwhelming support for this statement.

13. Bouchard and Wright, p. 135

14. Macdonald, p. 86

15. James, *Talks with Teachers*, p. 64

16. James, pp. 210-211

17. Alexander, *The Books of F. Matthias Alexander*, p. 416. See Lulie Westfeldt's discussion of Head-Neck-Back relations in her book, *F. Matthias Alexander: The Man and his Work.*

18. See Von Durckheim's book *Hara: The Vital Center in Man*, Chapter 5–The Practice of Right Posture.

19. Staring, pp. 25-26

20. Qtd. by Staring, p. 23

21. Ibid, p. 23

22. Qtd. by Staring, p.39

23. Ibid, p. 40

24. Alexander, *The Books of F. Matthias Alexander*, p. 420

25. Staring, p. 170

26. Staring, p. 40

27. James, pp. 192-193

28. James, p. 193

29. James, pp. 194-195

30. James, p. 187

31. Cohen, p. 93

32. Huxley, "The Education of an Amphibian" in *Tomorrow and Tomorrow and Tomorrow and other essays*, pp. 15-16

33. Ron Dennis, Personal Communication, Oct. 25, 2000

34. *Science and the Modern World*, p. 5

35. Sherrington, *Man on His Nature*, p. 153

36. Sherrington, *The Endeavor of Jean Fernel*, p. 89

37. In recent years, Dennis has suggested the notion of "skill" as a foundational formulation for posture-movement education. Dennis has characterized the achievements of Alexander and others in terms of their expansion of the possibilities for acquiring and improving the skills of body support and movement in everyday life. See Dennis' articles, "Primary Control and the Crisis in Alexander Technique Theory" and "Poise and the Art of Lengthening."

38. See Dennis' definition of the Alexander Technique in the first chapter of this book. See also his discussion of "un-exercise" at http://www.posturesense.com/FAQ.htm

Part II – Necessary Background
1. Ibn Paquda, qtd. in Rosten, p. 285

Chapter 5
1. Anonymous, qtd. in Macnab, p. 19

2. Brunnstrom, p.11

3. Qtd. in Smallheiser, p. 3

4. Kapandji, p. 20

5. Lumbar syndromes, 61.94%; cervical syndromes, 36.1%; thoracic syndromes, 1.96% according to Kramer, p. 13

6. Kramer, p. 18. Much of the discussion on the disc is indebted to Kramer's work.

7. Kramer, p. 26

8. See Kapandji, p. 40 and Kramer, pp. 28-29. Fennel and associates demonstrated these internal movements in their study, "Migration of the Nucleus Pulposus within the Intervertebral Disc during Flexion and Extension of the Spine" *Spine* 21 (23): pp. 2753-2757 (1996).

9. Kramer, p. 8. McKenzie (1990) points to research studies that support this notion of displacement of material inside the disc. See references on pp. 48, 204, and 206 of *The Cervical and Thoracic Spine.*

10. Cyriax, *The Slipped Disc*, pp. 74-75

11. Brunnstrom, p. 42

12. See "The Double Spiral Mechanism of the Voluntary Musculature of the Human Body," in Dart. This was originally published in *British Journal of Physical Medicine,* 13 (1946). Also see Kapandji, pp. 101 and 102. Implications of spirally-arranged musculature for posture-movement education are presented in Troup Mathew's article, "Blessed Helicity."

13. Dennis, "Poise and the Art of Lengthening"

Chapter 6

1. Melzack and Wall, p. 122

2. Ibid, p. 35

3. Ibid, pp. 41-47

4. Ibid, pp. 47-49

5. Ibid, pp. 124-127

6. Cyriax and Cyriax, *Illustrated Manual of Orthopaedic Medicine,* pp. 10-11

7. Robert P. Pula, writer/teacher of General Semantics (lecture notes)

8. "IASP Pain Terminology" from Merskey and Bogduk, *Classification of Chronic Pain*, pp. 209-214

9. See Melzack and Wall, pp. 222-239.

10. See Candace Pert's *The Chemistry of Emotion* for a firsthand account of the discovery of the endorphins and endorphin receptors. Rossi's *The Psychobiology of Mind-Body Healing* discusses the implications of the existence of these communication molecules.

11. Melzack and Wall, p. 402

12. The diagram and discussion are based on Alfred Korzybski's model of human perception/cognition presented in his article, "The Role of Language in the Perceptual Processes," in *Alfred Korzybski Collected Writings 1920-1950*, p. 683-720. This model is presented and discussed in *Drive Yourself Sane*.

13. Cyriax, *Textbook of Orthopaedic Medicine, Vol. I*, p. 569

Chapter 7

1. See Robert Fritz, *The Path of Least Resistance* and *Creating*.

2. William T. Powers, *Making Sense of Behavior: The Meaning of Control*, p. 7

3. The example of the driver staying in the lane is from *Making Sense of Behavior*, pp. 8-11.

4. A brief, non-technical introduction to Perceptual Control Theory is Powers' book *Making Sense of Behavior*. Also see Richard J. Robertson's article "Control Theory." Powers' *Living Control Systems I and II* and *Behavior: The Control of Perception* also contain many interesting articles. Other treatments of this important, paradigm-shifting approach to the human sciences include *Introduction to Modern Psychology: The Control-Theory View* by Richard J. Robertson and William T. Powers, Richard S. Marken's *Mind Readings: Experimental Studies of Purpose*, Philip J. Runkel's *Casting Nets and Testing Specimens* and Gary Cziko's *The Things We Do*.

5. Richard J. Robertson, "Control Theory," p. 170

6. See Runkel, p. 109 for another diagram of a negative feedback control loop. Runkel's chapter "Control Theory" in his book *Casting Nets and Testing Specimens* provides a brief, authoritative account of Perceptual Control Theory.

7. Robertson, op. cit.

8. See Powers' essay "Possible Levels of Perception and Control" in the appendix "Reference" of *Making Sense of Behavior*, pp. 135-152.

9. Robertson, op. cit., p. 171

10. Powers, *Making Sense of Behavior*, p. 55

11. Neev, pp. 9-13

12. Ford, p. 91

13. Wall, *Pain: The Science of Suffering*, p. 177

14. Wilfred Barlow, M.D., first discussed "postural homeostasis" in "Physical Education Research" in *More Talk of Alexander*, pp. 90-101, and later in *The Alexander Technique*, pp.79-82.

Part III – Therapy Solutions

1. Wall, *Pain: The Science of Suffering*, p. 100

Chapter 8

1. Waddell, pp. 10-11. The general categories of "simple backache," "nerve root pain," and "possible serious spinal pathology" is thoroughly presented in Waddell's Chapter 2, "Diagnostic Triage."

2. Ibid, p. 10

3. Ibid, p. 11

4. The notion of "red flag" situations and the list of questions is derived from Waddell, pp. 10-12.

5. *The Anatomy of Judgement*, pp. 138-139

6. Cyriax and Cyriax, *Illustrated Manual of Orthopaedic Medicine*, p. 23

7. See Mark Laslett, *Mechanical Diagnosis and Therapy: The Upper Limb*, Chapter 2, "Diagnosis", pp. 20-22.

8. Geoffrey D. Maitland "The Maitland Concept: Assessment, Examination, and Treatment by Passive Movement," in Twomey and Taylor, p. 137

9. Ibid, p. 138

10. Ibid, p. 138

11. Jacob and McKenzie, in Liebenson, p. 227

12. See Paula Van Wijmen, "The Use of Repeated Movements in The McKenzie Method of Spinal Examination." Also see Gary Jacob and Robin McKenzie, "Spinal Therapeutics Based On Responses To Loading."

13. Jacob and McKenzie, p. 225

14. Qtd. in Feyerabend, p. 194

Chapter 9

1. Previous circular models of pain reactions (common in the literature) have not explicitly traced feedback loops to the extent that this one does. See Paris; Cummings, et al.; and Waddell.

2. Waddell, pp. 225-228

3. Arthur Koestler, *The Act of Creation*, qtd. in Danysh, p. 79

4. Wall, *Pain: The Science of Suffering*, p. 48

5. Ibid, p. 34

6. Ibid, p. 36

7. Ibid, pp. 125-140

8. *Consciousness*, p. 235

9. Wall, p. 51

10. Ibid, pp. 49-51

11. Ibid, p. 52

12. Liebman, p. 38

13. McKenzie, *The Lumbar Spine*, pp. 22-24

14. Wall, p.145

15. Ibid

16. See Cummings, Crutchfield and Barnes, *Soft Tissue Changes in Contractures*, p. 3.

17. Ibid, pp. 3-5

18. Ibid, pp. 86, 105

19. Ibid, p. 113

20. McKenzie, *The Lumbar Spine*, pp. 11-12; Chapter 10, "The Dysfunction Syndrome," pp. 95-108

21. Cummings et al., pp. 72-110

22. *The Lumbar Spine*, Chapter 11, "The Derangement Syndrome"; *The Cervical and Thoracic Spine*, pp. 35-37

23. Cummings et al., pp. 113-114

24. See Kramer, pp. 28-29. Kramer placed asymmetrical pressures on lumbar disc specimens that had been removed from spines. His book provides measurements and photographs that demonstrate the movement of material within the disc. He reported that "Asymmetrical loading causes the nucleus pulposus [the inner gel portion] to move to an area of the disk which carries less load; forward bending causes it to move posteriorly, backward bending moves it anteriorly and lateral bending moves it to the opposite side" (p. 28). He concluded that "Postures of the spine which result in decentralization of the nucleus pulposus due to asym-

metrical loading of the intervertebral segment play an important role in the pathogenesis and in the prophylaxis of intervertebral disk disease" (p. 29).

25. McKenzie, *The Lumbar Spine*, p. 22. Also see *The Cervical and Thoracic Spine*, Chapter 7, "The Phenomenon of Pain Centralisation."

26. Research studies that explore the Centralization Phenomenon include: Donelson, Silva, and Murphy, "The Centralization Phenomenon: Its Usefulness in Evaluating and Treating Referred Pain"; Audrey Long, "The Centralization Phenomenon: Its Usefulness as a Predictor of Outcome in Conservative Treatment of Chronic Low Back Pain"; and Mark Werneke and others, "A Descriptive Study of the Centralization Phenomenon: A Prospective Analysis"; among other studies.

27. See Dr. Stephen Kuslich et al., "The Tissue Origin of Low Back Pain and Sciatica: a Report of Pain Response to Tissue Stimulation During Operations on the Lumbar Spine Using Local Anesthesia." Kuslich, a spine surgeon, explored the possible sources of back pain with research done on patients receiving back surgery. The patients got a local anesthetic that allowed them to remain conscious. Dr. Kuslich stimulated many anatomical structures around the site of each operation. Kuslich and his colleagues found that structures such as the joint capsules on either side, most ligaments of the spine, as well as the muscles of the back, seemed surprisingly insensitive. They also found that while the disc itself did not seem sensitive, the posterior (back) wall of the disc, especially the outer portion, did. Also especially sensitive was the adjoining posterior longitudinal ligament. Both of these structures produced back pain when stimulated. Stimulating the outer spinal covering (called the dura) along with the disc wall caused pain in the buttock and thigh. Kuslich could reproduce leg pain by stimulating the spinal nerve root. All of these structures receive stress during a disc derangement and will be affected in the order noted above as a derangement gets bigger. This could explain the pain pattern commonly seen during peripheralization. It does not seem implausible that these structures could also get relieved in the reverse order (centralization) with a derangement capable of getting smaller in size.

Also see Donelson, Aprill, Medcalf, and Grant, "A Prospective Study of Centralization of Lumbar and Referred Pain: A Predictor of Symptomatic Discs and Annular Competence." In this study, Dr. Ron Donelson and colleagues were able to show that those people whose symptoms centralized with repeated movement testing had problematic but intact discs as indicated by discograms. Those who did not respond well to repeated movements were less likely to have intact discs. Discography is a technique for visualizing the inside of a disc with x-ray. A radio-opaque dye gets injected into a disc. The spread of the dye and changes in its position in relation to movements can indicate the integrity of the disc. Discography injection can also produce or increase symptoms in problematic discs.

28. *The Cervical and Thoracic Spine*, pp. 22-23

29. *The Lumbar Spine*, Chapter 9, "The Postural Syndrome" and *The Cervical And Thoracic Spine*, Chapter 13, "The Cervical Postural Syndrome," Chapter 14, "Treatment of the Cervical Postural Syndrome," and the "Treatment" section of Chapter 25, "The Thoracic Spine"

30. See their article "Low Back and Referred Pain: Diagnosis and A Proposed New System of Classification."

31. Cummings, et al., pp. 127-145

32. See Sarno, *Healing Back Pain*.

33. Whatmore and Kohli, pp. 102-103

34. Garrett Hardin, *Filters Against Folly*, p. 58

35. Ellis, pp. 19-20

36. Ellis, p. 144

37. Arnold Glasow qtd. by Laurence J. Peter in *Peter's Quotations: Ideas for Our Time*, p. 286

Chapter 10

1. *The Touch of Healing*, p. 21

2. See Kay Thompson, D.D.S., *Therapeutic Uses of Language*.

3. These include a wide range of educational and/or healing practices, including acupressure, the Alexander Technique, Body Harmony, Continuum Movement, cranio-sacral therapy, the Feldenkrais Method, Ideokinesis, Jin Shin Jyutsu, massage, mindfulness meditation, myofascial release, Qigong, Rubenfeld Synergy, Rolfing, Sensory Awareness, Shiatsu, Simple Contact, the Trager Approach and Zero Balancing, among others. Mention here doesn't necessarily mean unqualified endorsement by me of the particular theory or practice associated with a discipline.

4. Ward, *The Brilliant Function of Pain*, p. 18

5. Ibid, pp. 30-31

6. Ibid, pp. 31, 32-33

7. Kodish and Kodish, p. 210

8. Ibid, p. 171

9. Ibid, p. 170

10. A version of this kind of figure is used by many healthcare professionals dealing with musculoskeletal pain.

11. Keyes, p. 141

12. Kodish and Kodish, p. 172

13. I derived the list of activities from the examination questionaire used by Robin McKenzie. Clinicians of many different schools of therapy use similar lists when questioning patients.

14. Keyes, p. 119

15. Kodish and Kodish, p. 173

16. These general rules of thumb (or back) are derived from the work of McKenzie and associates.

17. Gary Jacob, D.C., discusses some reasons for overemphasizing flexion in his article, "Specific Application of Movement and Positioning Technique to the Lumbar Spine, Considering Theoretical Formulation and Therapeutic Application."

18. Livingstone, p. 82

19. These exercises come from McKenzie's text, *The Lumbar Spine* and his self-care guide, *Treat Your Own Back.* You can find an accessible introduction to McKenzie's treatment approach in *7 Steps To A Pain-free Life.*

20. *The Lumbar Spine*, p. 18

21. Reinert's and Barge's writings are referenced in the informative article by Barrale et al., "Manipulative Management of Lumbar Disc Bulge."

22. *Textbook of Orthopaedic Medicine, Vol. I*, p. 535

23. McKenzie, "Re: Understanding Centralisation," p. 6

24. McKenzie and May, *The Human Extremities: Mechanical Diagnosis & Therapy*, p. 311

25. You can go to http://www.mckenziemdt.org/ on the World Wide Web to find a credentialed or diplomaed practitioner of McKenzie's

approach to mechanical diagnosis and therapy near you. In the United States you can call (800) 635-8380 for a referral. There are also practitioners of other approaches to activity-related therapy who may be able to help you.

26. The traffic light metaphor of green, red and yellow lights was created and developed as a guide for treatment by physical therapists Jean Duffy Rath and Wayne Rath. See Van Wijman, p. 25.

27. Cyriax, *The Slipped Disc*, p. 76

Part IV – Education Solutions

1. Alexander, *Articles and Lectures*, p. 198

Chapter 11

1. See Chapter 2, The Problem with 'Posture', and related notes 24, 25 and 26.

2. Goldthwait and others, p. 37. See pp. 32-37 for a discussion of general factors that enter into body mechanics. The book by Goldthwait et al. has long been out of print. You may be able to find it in a used book store. The region of motion where a factor-of-safety exists seems equivalent to what spine biomechanics researcher M.M. Punjabi calls the "neutral zone" of spinal motion ("The neutral zone is the initial portion of the [range of motion] during which spinal motion is produced against minimal internal resistance." [Julie M. Fritz et al, p. 890]) Punjabi refers to the end range area of motion as the "elastic zone" ("...the portion nearer to the end-range of movement that is produced against substantial internal resistence" [Ibid]). According to Punjabi, normal spinal stability depends upon the ability "to maintain the spinal neutral zones within physiological limits so that there is no neurological deficit, no major deformity, and no incapacitating pain" (Ibid, p. 891).

3. My analysis of exercise closely follows Alexander's arguments in his first book *Man's Supreme Inheritance* in *The Books of F. Matthias Alexander*. In particular, see Chapter II, "Primitive Remedies and Their Defects" and his discussion of the case of John Doe, pp. 19-23 and 61-63.

4. "Physical therapy, like any other discipline, has its share of dearly held beliefs. Perhaps none is stronger than the notion that static and dynamic postures are directly related to muscular strength. This is not true." (Barrett Dorko, "A Big Mistake.") See Dorko's article for "references and commentary from peer-reviewed literature [that] support [his] contention that strength and posture are unrelated."

5. As an example of this see Flowers' and Caputo's brief discussion of posture and spinal alignment in their book on strength training , pp. 15-16.

6. In their article, "Spinal Stabilization Exercise Program," Jerry Hyman, D.C., and Craig Liebenson, D.C., review this approach to spinal rehabilitation and posture-movement education. They state a basic "rule for training the 'failed back': Find the painfree range of motion or functional range" (p. 294). This accords with Goldthwait's emphasis on the factor–of–safety motion.

7. See Jill Coleman's book, *Water Yoga* (which can be used in and out of the water). Also see Kenneth Cohen's, *The Way of Qigong.* Aat Dekker's article, "The Tao of Korzybski?" provides a rare and necessary formulation of Tai Chi and related practices (Qigong) in terms of 'western' neurophysiology and scientific humanist philosophy. For another treatment of Tai Chi that avoids questionable metaphysics, see the work of William C. C. Chen, *Body Mechanics of Tai Chi Chuan.*

8. See "Can An Educational Booklet Change Behavior and Pain In Chronic Low Back Pain Patients" by B.E. Udermann et al.

9. This notion, seen within the context of Perceptual Control Theory, qualifies as what Edmund C. Berkeley called a "Thousand Horsepower Idea." Korzybski was perhaps the first to explore the notion of mapping in relation to nervous system functioning, language and behavior in *Science and Sanity* (1933*)*. Somewhat later (1943) related notions were taken up by Kenneth Craik in his discussion of internal models in the brain in *The Nature of Explanation* (see the entry under his name in R. L. Gregory, *The Oxford Companion to the Mind*). A recent work on cognitive maps is that of Ervin Laszlo and others, *Changing Visions.* You can find an introduction to Korzybski's practical approach to using these notions in everyday life in *Drive Yourself Sane.*

10. Information on PostureSense® classes is available at www.posturesense.com

11. For further information on the Alexander Technique and referrals to certified AT teachers in your area, you can phone the American Society for the Alexander Technique (AmSAT) at (800) 473-0620 or 413-584-2359. You can also get information and a list of certified teachers at the AmSAT website, http://www.alexandertech.com/ You can also write to AmSAT, P.O. Box 60008, Florence, MA 01062 for further information, a certified teachers list and a booklist .

12. Pula, p. 64

13. An old limerick warns of the problems associated with spastic self-preoccupation:

The centipede was happy quite
Until the toad in fun,
Said, "Pray, which leg goes after which?"
This led his brain to such a pitch,
He lay distracted in a ditch
Considering how to run.

Chapter 12

1. Langer, *Mindfulness*, p. 1

2. *Drive Yourself Sane*, pp. 36-48

3. Much of the material in this and the next section comes from Chapter 8 of *Drive Yourself Sane*, "Non-verbal Awareness," and from an article of mine, "Emptying Your Cup: Non-verbal Awareness and General Semantics" published in *ETC: A Review of General Semantics*.

4. From Wendell Johnson's book entitled, appropriately enough, *Your Most Enchanted Listener* (p. 5)

5. Three excellent books about this discipline are Charles Brooks' *Sensory Awareness: The Rediscovery of Experiencing*, Betty Winkler Keane's *Sensing: Letting Yourself Live*, and Carola Speads' *Breathing: The ABC's*. You can also find more at the Sensory Awareness Foundation website at http://www.sensoryawareness.org/index.html

6. "Charlotte Schuchardt Read on Sensory Awareness" from videotaped interview with Louise Boedeker (April, 1999) in *Sensory Awareness Foundation Newsletter*, Summer 2000. Available at http://www.sensoryawareness.org/newsletter/summer00/charlotte.html

7. See "On Conscious Abstracting and a Consciousness of Abstracting" (Part I) and (Part II) by Milton Dawes. Also see his article, "The Wedge of Consciousness: A Self-Monitoring Device" located on the Institute of General Semantics website at http://www.general-semantics.org/ Click on the Basics button.

8. From newspaper article (now lost) in *The Baltimore Sun*, dated sometime in the late 1990s

9. Now neuroscientists consider the notion of maps in the brain a standard part of their science. See the article "Localization of Brain Function and Cortical Maps" in R. L. Gregory's *The Oxford Companion to the Mind*. See also Note 8 for Chapter 11.

10. Sacks, *The Man Who Mistook His Wife For A Hat*, pp. 55-58

11. Reported in Barlow's *The Alexander Technique* (pp.17-18). The original study was published in 1947 as "An Investigation Into Kinaesthesia" in *British Journal of Physical Medicine* 10 (81) and reprinted in Barlow's book, *More Talk of Alexander*, in Chapter 8, "Physical Education Research."

12. Montagu, *Touching*, p. 401

13. See Hanna's book *Somatics.*

14. Oliver Sacks, in an article on "Nothingness" in the *Oxford Companion to the Mind*, writes: "Blockage to the spinal cord or the great limb plexuses can produce an identical situation [to that of brain injury], even though the brain is intact but deprived of the information from which it might form an image...Indeed it can be shown by measuring potentials in the brain during spinal or regional blocks that there is a dying away of activity in the corresponding part of the cerebral representation of the 'body-image'...Similar annihilations may be brought out peripherally, either through nerve or muscle damage in a limb, or by simply enclosing the limb in a cast, which by its mixture of immobilization and encasement may temporarily bring neural traffic and impulses to a halt" (pp. 564-565).

15. *A Leg To Stand On*, p. 98

16. "Dr. Michael Merzenich and his collaborators...have shown that...brain pathways for registering touch sensations are not hard wired, but remain fluid in adulthood." (Montagu, p. 289)

17. *A Leg To Stand On*, p. 150

18. From the song "Dancing With Myself," words and music (1980) by Billy Idol and Tony James, on the album *Billy Idol*

Chapter 13

1. Alexander referred to this as "unreliable sensory appreciation."

2. The title of Binkley's book on the Alexander Technique, wherein he gives an account of his lessons with F. M. Alexander

3. Lulu Sweigard detailed her work in body mechanics education, which she called "ideokinesis," in her book, *Human Movement Potential*. She was a student of Mabel Ellsworth Todd, another pioneer in the field of posture-movement education, whose own book is called *The Thinking Body*.

4. Call 715-284-5381 to order the Spinatrac™ posture tool for $15.90 with shipping.

5. You can learn a great deal about chairs, sitting and body use from Galen Cranz's book, *The Chair.* Cranz, an Alexander Technique teacher and professor of the sociology of architecture, gives not only a fascinating history of chairs but also provides helpful suggestions for what she calls "body-conscious design."

6. See A.C. Mandal, "Balanced Sitting Posture On Forward Sloping Seat."

7. *The Slipped Disc*, p. 79

8. "...the first doctor to advocate a lumbar convexity to the chair to support [the] lumbar spine in lordosis was Taylor of New York in 1864." (Cyriax, *The Slipped Disc*, p. 79)

9. Williams, Hawley, Van Wijman, McKenzie, "A Comparison of the Effects of Two Sitting Postures on Back and Referred Pain"

10. See Egill Snorrason's article, "Exercise for Healthy Persons," pp. 901-903, published in 1965.

11. McKenzie, *The Lumbar Spine*, pp. 86-87; *The Cervical Spine*, pp. 161-163

12. *The Cervical Spine*, pp. 162-163

13. See www.posturesense.com, "About PostureSense®."

14. Tucker, *Active Alerted Posture*

15. See Kendall and McCreary, *Muscles: Testing and Function. Third Edition*, Chapter 8, "Muscle Function in Relation to Posture," pp. 269-316. This chapter provides excellent detailed photos and descriptions of a variety of static postural faults. McKenzie describes a couple of typical standing slumps in *The Lumbar Spine*, pp. 90-91.

16. I have derived the movement experiments for standing balance from Moshe Feldenkrais, *Awareness Through Movement*, pp. 77-78. Feldenkrais studied the Alexander Technique when he was formulating his own system of posture-movement education.

17. See Kenneth J. Cohen, *The Way of Qigong.* In this well-written and scholarly book, Cohen advocates traditional notions of Chinese medicine. This includes the theory of Qi (pronounced chee), an unseen vital substance containing the 'essence' of life. Cohen sees this theory as complementary with modern science. The phenomena that Cohen writes about may have potential significance for health. Many of the practices that Cohen teaches appear to have value. How to talk about and explain them remains an important question. I am not sure that the theory of Qi

has any more usefulness for modern biology and medicine than the now abandoned theory of phlogiston has for chemistry (see Conant, *On Understanding Science*, pp. 81-101).

18. Cohen, p. 86

19. Cohen, p. 96

20. Alexander's earliest known writings from 1894 to 1908 concerned "vocal and respiratory re-education." See his *Articles and Lectures.*

21. *Essentials of Body Mechanics*, p. 56

22. Austin and Ausubel's research paper can be found in *The Alexander Technique: Published Research,* available from the American Society for the Alexander Technique.

23. See *Freedom to Change* by Frank Pierce Jones, pp. 21-22.

24. Beckett Howorth, M.D., "Dynamic Posture," Journal of the American Medical Association, Aug. 24, 1946, p. 1402

25. "In animal studies the term 'reafference' has been used to describe the neural excitation that follows sensory stimulation produced by voluntary movements of the animal doing the sensing. The principle of reafference applies in teaching the Alexander Technique whenever the pupil is encouraged to move voluntarily while the teacher facilitates some aspect of the anti-gravity response" (Jones, p.157).

26. www.posturesense.com, "About PostureSense®"

27. Jones, pp. 69-70

28. See *The Use of the Self,* Chapter I, "The Evolution of a Technique" in *The Books of F.M. Alexander.* In the last few pages of this chapter, Alexander describes the steps I've noted here as a way of working—thinking in activity—that you can apply to anything you do. (pp. 427-429)

Chapter 14

1. See the Web page of OSHA, the Occupational Safety & Health Administration, http://www.osha-slc.gov/SLTC/ergonomics

2. *The Chair*, p. 158. Cranz provides recommendations for chairs and chair use that I generally endorse with this exception—I often advise the use of lumbar supports. See Chapter 13, herein, on Supported Sitting.

3. See Note 6, Chapter 13.

4. McKenzie, *The Lumbar Spine*, pp. 91-92

5. McKenzie, *The Cervical Spine*, pp. 167-168

6. For sitting, Mandal recommends a desk height measuring one half of your standing height and a chair height reaching one third of it ("Balanced sitting posture on forward sloping seat"). He also recommends sloping desk surfaces that tilt the work up towards the user.

7. See article "Spinal Overload" published in *The Back Letter.*

8. See Pheasant and Stubbs's, "Back Pain in Nurses: Epidemiology and Risk Assessment." For a general treatment of occupational injuries, see *Work-Related Musculoskeletal Disorders.*

9. Wassell et al., "A Prospective Study of Back Belts for Prevention of Back Pain and Injury."

Chapter 15

1. In his 1975 book, *The Gravity Guiding System*, Robert Mannat Martin, M.D., wrote, "[Man] is compelled to live in a potentially backache-producing environment of relentless, unidirectional gravity. However, through his ability to employ postural variety, he can live successfully and comfortably in such an environment. *Planned and properly guided postural exchange is the prime tool for prevention and correction of common backache and many, many other physical problems*" (p. 7). Martin advocated the varied use of six basic postures: the erect, horizontal, flexed, extended, brachiated (hanging by arms) and inverted (upside-down) positions.

2. Cranz, p. 185

3. I've based this principle on the work of many individuals. John M. Barbis, a professor of physical therapy at Thomas Jefferson University, expressed the underlying viewpoint well in his article "Prevention and Management of Low Back Pain." Here he emphasized the importance of "balancing flexion and extension" and "the prevention of prolonged loading or repetitive motions in one direction." (pp. 66-67)

4. McKenzie, *The Cervical and Thoracic Spine*, pp. 116-119

5. Stoddard, pp. 69, 73

6. My recommendations on when to consult your physician are based on American College of Sports Medicine guidelines (Bazley, p. 45).

7. Bazely points out that "The prescription of '3 to 4 times per week, 30 to 40 minutes per session' has become known as 'the fitness formula' and is the frequency and duration of exercise needed to stimulate an

aerobic effect and help prevent disease. It will take approximately 11 to 12 weeks to reach the desired aerobic level, and exercise must be maintained over a lifetime in order to continue to maintain the aerobic and protective benefit" (p. 45). Recent research indicates that this fitness formula is not as fixed as perhaps once thought. Shorter periods of time (10 minutes or less) that add up to the 30 or 40 minute total may provide substantial benefits. "Walking bouts of only five minutes—when added up to 30 minutes per day on most days of the week—can improve cardiovascular health and body composition, according to a study published last year [1999] in *Preventive Medicine*. Stair climbing, done for 2 1/4 minutes, six times a day, conferred 'considerable health benefits on previously sendentary young women,' this same journal reported in April [2000]." (Krucoff)

8. "Got No Time For Serious Fitness Training? The Long and Short of It; Exercise: Researchers now say that little 'sparks' of activity throughout the day can offer health benefits." *Los Angeles Times*, 12/04/00, pp. S1, S8

9. See the website of Grand Master William C.C. Chen for a listing of teachers certified by him: http://www.williamccchen.com/ Also see the T'ai Chi Chih homepage for information about this simplified Tai Chi exercise form which I have found useful and easy to learn: http://www.taichichih.org/index.htm Also see the book by Master Justin Stone. You might also find useful the related practice of Zhan Zhuang (pronounced "Jan Jong"). Zhan Zhuang, a standing meditation/exercise, translates from Chinese as "standing like a tree." See Master Lam Kam Chuen's book *The Way of Energy* and his website http://www.chi-kung.org/chikung-e/index.htm

10. *Fitness Without Stress*, p. 11

11. "The art of combining relaxation with activity has been invented and reinvented by the teachers of every kind of psycho-physical skill" (Aldous Huxley, "The Education of an Amphibian," in *Tomorrow and Tomorrow and Tomorrow*, p. 18).

12. Dart, *Skill and Poise*, p. 8

13. See Trager and Guadagno.

14. "Rest means rest from function or weight bearing, not from movement. Movement must be maintained" (Mennel, p. 126).

15. Discussed in the book *EEVeTeCh* by Dr. Rob Roy McGregor. The letters EEVeTeCh stand for five basic factors that McGregor suggests

need to be addressed in order to reduce and prevent sports injuries: E – Equipment, E – Environment, Ve –Velocity, Te – Technique, and C – Conditioning.

16. "Of all the practices known to be associated with good health, sleep is the most fundamental. The most basic step you can take to improve your health is to figure out how much sleep you need and to see that you get it" (Hobson, *The Chemistry of Conscious States*, p. 226).

17. In an interview with Selye in Denis Brian's *Genius Talk: Conversations with Nobel Scientists and Other Luminaries* (p. 271)

Conclusion
1. Murrow's Law in Peter, *Peter's People,* p. 204

Chapter 16
1. Waddell, pp. 45-46

2. Waddell, p. 83

3. "How Quackery Sells," p. 14

4. Long, "The Centralization Phenomenon: Its Usefulness as a Predictor of Outcome in Conservative Treatment of Chronic Low Back Pain (a Pilot Study)"

5. Fisher, "Early Experiences of a Multidisciplinary Pain Management Programme"

6. Snook et al., "The Reduction of Chronic Nonspecific Low Back Pain Through the Control of Early Morning Lumbar Flexion: A Randomized Controlled Trial"

7. Manipulative treatment cannot cure disease. As a form of mechanical therapy, it seems especially useful when self-treatment measures have proven insufficient. Then, in the cases that require it, manipulation—passive movements to the joints applied by the therapist—can result in improved symptoms and increased mobility and allow a person to successfully proceed with self-treatment. Manipulation can be unsafe and promote dependency when not preceeded by repeated movement testing and preliminary self-treatment.

Unfortunately, some chiropractors have fabricated the view that their profession has some special claim to doing manipulation. They are presently lobbying many state legislatures to prevent physical therapists from performing manipulation. In actuality, while manipulation has been used for centuries, the system of chiropractic was founded relatively recently, in the 1890s, on the basis of what many medical professionals—and even some chiropractors—now consider exaggerated claims and questionable evidence.

Manipulative treatment has often, although certainly not always, been abused by a significant number of chiropractors. Stephen Barrett, M.D., discusses and documents questionable chiropractic practices in his article, "The Spine Salesmen." Also see the article, "Chiropractic: Does the Bad Outweigh the Good?" by Samuel Homola, D.C. and the books, *Inside Chiropractic* by Homola and *Chiropractic: The Victim's Perspective* by George Magner.

Many chiropractors continue to base their work upon scientifically-implausible theories and practices. Fortunately, some chiropractors question and seek to move beyond them. Some chiropractors practice some form of posture-movement therapy and/or education, as discussed in this book. Some belong to the National Association for Chiropractic Medicine, an organization which has renounced "the historical chiropractic philosophy that subluxation [a vague and medically unaccepted diagnosis, as many chiropractors use it] is the cause of disease" (Barrett, p. 167). Responsible chiropractors acknowledge the paucity of scientific research on the usefulness of manipulative treatment and are working with their colleagues in other fields to correct this situation.

8. Esteemed spine researcher Alf Nachemson, M.D., writes "The direction from today's available studies is fairly clear: examine, encourage, exercise, pay attention to psychosocial deterrents to function, and involve the workplace in the rehabilitation of those with work disability...Work can actually be remedial...Politicians, union leaders, and patients must all understand this life-saving message. An early disability pension endangers your life." (A. Nachemson. 2000. Preface. In *Neck and Back Pain: The Scientific Evidence of Causes, Diagnosis and Treatment*. Edited by A. Nachemson and E. Jonsson, xi. Philadelphia: Williams & Wilkins. Qtd. in "Life-Saving Prescription," *The Back Letter*)

9. Huxley, p. 31

10. Arsenault, pp. 231-232

11. Arsenault, p. 234. You can contact The Moving to Learn Society at 4246 Peachtree Rd. #6, Atlanta, GA 30319

12. *Growing Young*, p. 2. Montagu once said "The idea is to die young as late as possible." William T. Powers had something similar in view when he said "I have finally figured out what I want to be when I grow up: dead." (*Making Sense of Behavior*, p. ii)

13. In regard to the unity and inseparability of 'mind' and 'body', Montagu wrote "...mind and brain are definitely not synonyms...the development of the human mind depends on contact with other human beings in a human society...Mind represents the expression of the social organization of the nervous elements of the whole body...Regard every part of your nervous system in its total relations as comprising your mind...no amount of manipulation would cause your little finger to perform the tricks necessary in the playing of the piano, for example, if some sort of nervous organization had not occurred within it. The nerve structures in your little finger are as necessary as those in your brain. For the purpose of piano playing they are both indispensable parts of your mind. The pianist's fingers are culturally quite as highly organized as his brain must be in order to read the music which his fingers help to produce. He has the score, literally, 'at his finger tips.' " (*On Being Intelligent*, p. 4-9)

14. "...every bit of relevant evidence indicates that infirmities and breakdowns are much less likely to occur in those who have retained a youthful spirit than in those who have succumbed to the self-fulfilling prophecy of aging, and have aged in accordance with what is ritually expected of them...limberness diminishes with reduced movement...ideas, feelings, playfulness also diminish with reduced expression. The diminished become quiet, withdrawn, unexpressive...it is not the years that diminish us. It is the way we have learned to live them, giving up a little of our true selves at each step." (Montagu, *Growing Young*, pp. 199-203)

15. See the works of Alexander, Brooks, Edwards, Feldenkrais, Hanna Montagu and Sharaf.

Bibliography

Abercrombie, M. L. J. 1960. *The anatomy of judgement*. London: Penguin Books.

Acute back pain benign but frequently persistent. 1999. *The Back Letter* 14 (6):63.

Ackerknecht, Erwin H. 1982. *A Short History of Medicine*. Revised Edition. Baltimore: The Johns Hopkins University Press.

Alexander, F. Matthias. 1997. *The Books of F. Matthias Alexander.* New York: IRDEAT. (Available from Institute for Research, Development and Education in the Alexander Technique, 74 MacDougal St. NY, NY 10012)

————. 1995. *Articles and lectures: Articles, published letters and lectures on the F. M. Alexander Technique.* Notes by Jean M. O. Fischer. London: Mouritz.

American Chiropractic Association (ACA). 1987. ACA policies on public health and related matters: Promotion of good postural awareness. Available at http://www.amerchiro.org/index.html

American Society for the Alexander Technique. (North American Society for Teachers of the Alexander Technique). 1997. *The Alexander Technique: Published research.* Northhampton, MA: AmSAT Books.

Armstrong, H., A.M. Jones and D.H. Rosenbaum. 1992. Nonoperative management of herniated nucleus pulposus: Patient selection by the extension sign—Long-term follow-up. *Orthopaedic Review* XXI (2).

Arsenault, Michele. 1998. *Moving to learn: A classroom guide to understanding and using good body mechanics.* Atlanta, GA: The Moving to Learn Society, Inc.

Austin, John H.M. and Pearl Ausubel. August 1992. Enhanced respiratory muscular functioning in normal adults after lessons in proprioceptive musculoskeletal education without exercise. *Chest* 102:486-490.

Barbis, John M. 1992. Prevention and management of low back pain. In *Prevention practice: Strategies for physical therapy and occupational therapy,* ed. Jeffrey Rothman and Ruth Levine, 63-73. Philadelphia: W.B. Saunders.

Barlow, Wilfred. 1973, 1990. *The Alexander Technique: How to use your body without stress.* Rochester, VT: Healing Arts Press.

Barlow, Wilfred, ed. 1978. *More talk of Alexander:Aspects of the Alexander principle.* London:Victor Gollancz Ltd.

Barrale, Ralph; et al. 1989. Manipulative management of lumbar disc bulge. *Chiropractic Technique* 1 (3): 79-87.

Barrett, Stephen. 1993. The Spine Salesmen. In *The health robbers: A close look at quackery in America*, ed. Stephen Barrett, M.D. and William T. Jarvis, Ph.D, 161-190. Buffalo: Prometheus Books.

Barrett, Stephen and William T. Jarvis, eds. 1993. *The health robbers: A close look at quackery in America..* Buffalo: Prometheus Books.

Bazley, Robert D. 1992. Promoting health through exercise. In *Prevention practice: Strategies for physical therapy and occupational therapy,* ed. Jeffrey Rothman and Ruth Levine, 36-59. Philadelphia: W.B. Saunders.

Berkeley, Edmund C. 1966. *A guide to mathematics for the intelligent nonmathematician.* New York: Simon and Schuster.

Bigos, S, O. Bowyer , G. Braen , et al. 1994. *Acute low back problems in adults. Clinical practice guideline no. 14.* AHCPR Publication No. 95-0642. Rockville, MD: Agency for Health Care Policy and Research, Public Health Service, U.S. Department of Health and Human Services.

Boden, Scott D., et al. March 1990. Abnormal magnetic-resonance scans of the lumbar spine in asymptomatic subjects. *Journal of Bone and Joint Surgery* 72 (3).

Bouchard, Ed and Ben Wright. 1997. *Kinesthetic ventures: Informed by the work of F.M. Alexander, Stanislavski, Peirce & Freud.* Ed. Michael Protzel. Chicago: MESA Press.

Brian, Denis. 1995. *Genius talk: Conversations with Nobel scientists and other luminaries.* New York: Plenum Press.

Brooks, Charles V.W. 1974. *Sensory awareness: The rediscovery of experiencing.* New York: The Viking Press.

Brunnstrom, Signe. 1979. *Clinical kinesiology.* Seventh Revised Printing. Revision by Ruth Dickinson. Philadelphia: F.A. Davis.

Burmeister, Alice with Tom Monte. 1997. *The touch of healing.* New York: Bantam.

Caplan, Deborah. 1987. *Back trouble: A new approach to prevention and recovery.* Gainesville, FL: Triad Publishing.

Carey, Timothy S. 1999. Recurrence and care seeking after acute back pain: Results of a long-term follow-up study. *Med Care* 37 (2): 157-164.

Chen, William C. C. 1973. *Body mechanics of Tai Chi Chuan.* New York: William C. C. Chen.

Cherkin, Daniel C., Richard A. Deyo, Kimberly Wheeler and Marcia A. Ciol. 1994. Physician variation in diagnostic testing for low back pain. *Arthritis & Rheumatism* 37 (1): 15-24.

Chuen, Lam Kam. 1991. *The way of energy: Mastering the Chinese art of internal strength with chi kung exercise.* New York: Simon & Schuster.

Clinical information from the international family medicine literature. 1999. *American Family Physician* 59 (7): 2000-2001.

Cohen, Kenneth S. 1997. *The way of qigong: The art and science of Chinese energy healing.* New York: Ballantine.

Coleman, Jill. 1996,1998. *WaterYoga: Water-assisted postures and stretches for flexibility and well-being.* Owings Mills, MD: Eglantine Press.

Conable, Barbara and William Conable. 1995. *How to learn the Alexander Technique: A manual for students.* Third Edition. Columbus, OH: Andover Press.

Conant, James B. 1951. *On understanding science: an historical approach.* New York: New American Library.

Corsini, Raymond J. and Alan J. Auerback, eds. 1996,1998. *Concise encyclopedia of psychology.* Second Ed., Abridged. New York: John Wiley & Sons.

Cranz, Galen. 1998. *The chair: Rethinking culture, body, and design.* New York: W. W. Norton.

Cummings, Gordon S., Carolyn A. Crutchfield and Marylou R. Barnes. 1983. *Soft tissue changes in contractures. Orthopedic Physical Therapy Series, Vol. I.* Atlanta, GA: Stokesville Publishing Co.

Cyriax, James and Patricia Cyriax. 1983. *Illustrated manual of orthopaedic medicine.* London: Butterworths.

Cyriax, James. 1980. *The slipped disc.* Third Edition. New York: Charles Scribner's Sons.

————. 1978. *Textbook of orthopaedic medicine: Volume one — Diagnosis of soft tissue lesions.* Seventh Edition. London: Baillière Tindall.

Cziko, Gary. 2000. *The things we do: Using the lessons of Bernard and Darwin to understand the what, how, and why of our behavior.* Cambridge, MA: MIT Press.

Danysh, Joseph. 1974. *Stop without quitting.* San Francisco: International Society for General Semantics.

Dart, Raymond. N.d. *Skill and poise: A selection of writings of Raymond Arthur Dart.* Ed. Alexander Murray. U.S. paperback edition.

Dawes, Milton. 1999-2000. On conscious abstracting and a consciousness of abstracting, Part II. *ETC: A review of general semantics* 56 (4): 473-477.

————. 1999. On conscious abstracting and a consciousness of abstracting, Part I. *ETC: A review of general semantics* 56 (3): 351-356.

Dekker, Aat. 1995. The Tao of Korzybski? (An amalgamation of two papers: "The Tao of Korzybski" and "Tai Chi Chuan and Health (Including Sanity)." Ed. Robert P. Pula. *General Semantics Bulletin* 62

Delitto, A., M.T. Cibulka, R.E. Erhard, R.W. Bowling and J.A.Tenhula. 1993. Evidence for an extension-mobilization category in acute low back syndrome: A prescriptive validation pilot study. *Physical Therapy* 73 (4): 216-223.

Dennis, Ronald J. 1999a. Functional reach improvement in normal older women after Alexander Technique instruction. *Journal of Gerontology* 54A (1): M8-M11.

————. 1999b. Primary control and the crisis in Alexander Technique theory. *American Society for the Alexander Technique News* 45 (Summer 1999).

————.1991. Poise and the art of lengthening. http://www.neckfree.com/poise.htm

Deyo, Richard A. 1998. Low back pain. *Scientific American* August: 49-53.

Donelson , R., C. Aprill, R. Medcalf, and W. Grant. 1997. A prospective study of centralization of lumbar and referred pain: A predictor of symptomatic discs and annular competence. *Spine* 22 (10).

Donelson, R.,W. Grant, et al. 1991. Pain response to saggital end-range spinal motion: A multi-centered, prospective, randomized trial. *Spine* 16 (6): 206-212.

Donelson, Ronald, G. Silva, K. Murphy. 1990. The centralization phenomenon: Its usefulness in evaluating and treating referred pain. *Spine* 15 (3).

Dorko, Barrett. 2000. A big mistake. At http://www.barrettdorko.com/a_big_mistake.htm

———. 1996. *Shallow dive: Essays on the craft of manual care.* Thorofare, NJ: Slack.

Edwards, Paul. 1967. Reich, Wilhelm. In *The encyclopedia of philosophy.* Ed. Paul Edwards, 104-115. New York: Macmillan & The Free Press.

Ellis, Albert. 1988. *How to stubbornly refuse to make yourself miserable about anything yes anything!* Secaucus, NJ: Lyle Stuart Inc.

Feldenkrais, Moshe. 1972,1977. *Awareness through movement: Health exercises for personal growth.* New York: Harper & Row.

Fennell, A.J., A.P. Jones, D.W.L. Hukins. 1996. Migration of the nucleus pulposus within the intervertebral disc during flexion and extension of the spine. *Spine* 21 (23): 2753-275. Abstract by Ron Bybee.1997. *The McKenzie Institute USA Journal* 5 (1): 46.

Fenton, Jack Vinten. 1973. *Practical movement control: A sound method for developing good habits of body movement, control and poise in young people.* Boston: Plays, Inc.

Feyerabend, Paul. 1999. *Conquest of abundance: A tale of abstraction versus the richness of being.* Ed. Bert Terpstra. Chicago: The University of Chicago Press.

Fisher, Keren. 1988. Early experiences of a multidisciplinary pain management programme. *Holistic Medicine* 3 (1): 47-56.

Flowers, Brandon and Rick Caputo. 1999. *Where the rubber meets the road: Dynamic strength training with elastic resistance tubing.* Pasadena, CA: The Dynamic Advantage.

Ford, Edward E. 1993. *Freedom from stress.* Revised and expanded edition. Scottsdale, AZ: Brandt Publishing.

Fritz, Julie M., Richard E. Erhard, Brian F. Hagen. 1998. Segmental instability of the lumbar spine. *Physical Therapy* 78 (8): 889-896.

Fritz, Robert. 1991. *Creating.* New York: Fawcett Columbine.

———. 1984. *The path of least resistence: Principles for creating what you want to create.* Salem, MA: Stillpoint Publishing Company.

Garlick, David. 1990. *The lost sixth sense: A medical scientist looks at the Alexander Technique.* Laboratory for Musculoskeletal and Postural Research – School of Physiology and Pharmacology, The University of New South Wales.

Gelb, Michael J. 1995. *Body learning: An introduction to the Alexander Technique*. Second Edition. New York: Henry Holt.

Goldthwait, Joel E, Lloyd T. Brown, Loring T. Swaim and John G. Kuhns. 1934,1952. *Essentials of body mechanics in health and disease*. Fifth Edition. Philadelphia: J. B. Lippincott.

Greene, Dana. Fall 1996. Abstracts that discourage treatment based on imaging results alone. *The McKenzie Institute, USA Journal* 4 (4).

Gregory, Richard L., with the assistance of O. L. Zangwill. 1987. *The Oxford companion to the mind*. New York: Oxford University Press.

Haldeman, Scott. 1980. *Modern developments in the principles and practice of chiropractic*. New York: Appleton-Century-Crofts.

Hanna, Thomas. 1988. *Somatics: Reawakening the mind's control of movement, flexibility, and health*. Reading, MA: Addison-Wesley.

Hardin, Garrett. 1985. *Filters against folly: How to survive despite economists, ecologists, and the merely eloquent*. New York: Viking.

Hobson, J. Allan. 1999. *Consciousness*. New York: Scientific American Library.

———. *The chemistry of conscious states: How the brain changes its mind*. Boston: Little, Brown and Company.

Homola, Samuel. 2001. Chiropractic: Does the bad outweigh the good? *Skeptical Inquirer* 25 (1): 50-53.

———.1999. *Inside chiropractic: A patient's guide*. Buffalo, NY: Prometheus Books.

Howorth, Beckett. Dynamic posture. *Journal of the American Medical Association* 131 (17) 1946: 1398-1404.

Hyman, Jerry and Craig Liebenson. 1996. Spinal stabilization exercise program. In *Rehabilitation of the spine: A practitioner's manual*, ed. Craig Liebenson, 293-317. Baltimore: Williams & Wilkins.

Huxley, Aldous. 1956. The education of an amphibian. In *Tomorrow and tomorrow and tomorrow and other essays*, 1-32. New York. Harper and Brothers.

Idol, Billy. 1982. *Billy Idol*. Performed by Phil Feit, Billy Idol, Steve Missal, Steve Stevens. EMD/Crysalis compact disc.

Jacob, Gary. 1999. Specific application of movement and positioning techniques to the lumbar spine, considering theoretical formulation and therapeutic application. *The McKenzie Journal* 7 (2).

Jacob, Gary and Robin McKenzie. 1996. Spinal therapeutics based on responses to loading. In *Rehabilitation of the spine: A practitioner's manual*,
ed. Craig Liebenson, 225-252. Baltimore: Williams & Wilkins.

James, William. 1900. *Talks to teachers on psychology: And to students on
some of life's ideals.* New York: Henry Holt and Company.

Jarvis, William T. and Stephen Barrett. 1993. How quackery sells: Clinical
tricks of the supersalesman. In *The health robbers: A close look at quackery
in America*, ed. Stephen Barrett, M.D. and William T. Jarvis, Ph.D., 1-22.
Buffalo: Prometheus Books.

Jayson, Malcolm I.V., ed. 1987. *The lumbar spine and back pain.* Third
Edition. Edinburgh: Churchill Livingstone.

Johnson, Wendell. 1956. *Your most enchanted listener.* New York: Harper
& Row. Reprinted by the International Society for General Semantics, San
Francisco.

Jones, Frank Pierce. 1998. *Collected writings on the Alexander Technique.*
Ed. Theodore Dimon and Richard Brown. Cambridge, MA: Alexander Technique Archives, Inc.

————. 1997. *Freedom to change: The development and science of the Alexander Technique.* 3d. ed. (Formerly *Body awareness in action*, 1976).
London: Mouritz.

Kamenetz, Herman L. 1980. History of Massage. In *Manipulation, traction and massage.* Second Edition. Ed. Joseph B. Rogoff. Baltimore, MD: Williams & Wilkins.

Kapandji, I.A. 1974. *The physiology of the joints: Annotated diagrams of the mechanics of the human joints. Volume 3—The trunk and the vertebral column.*
Edinburgh: Churchill Livingstone.

Keane, Betty Winkler. 1979. *Sensing: Letting yourself live.* San Francisco: Harper
& Row.

Kelly, George A. 1963, 1955. *A theory of personality: The psychology of personal
constructs.* New York: W. W. Norton.

Keyes, Kenneth S., Jr. 1979, 1950. *How to develop your thinking ability.* New York:
McGraw-Hill.

Kendall, Florence P. and Elizabeth Kendall McCreary. 1983. *Muscles: Testing and
function.* Third Edition. Baltimore: Williams & Wilkins.

Kilby, J., M. Stigant and A. Roberts. Sept. 1990. The reliability of back pain assessment by physiotherapists, using a "McKenzie Algorithm." *Physiotherapy* 76 (9): 579-
583.

Kodish, Bruce I. 1998. Emptying your cup: Non-verbal awareness and general semantics. *Etc.: A review of general semantics* 55 (1) Spring: 16-29.

Kodish, Bruce I. and Susan Presby Kodish. 2001. *Drive yourself sane: Using the uncommon sense of general semantics.* Revised Second Edition. Pasadena, CA: Extensional Publishing.

Kodish, Susan Presby, ed. 1998. *Developing sanity in human affairs.* Contributions to the study of mass media and communications, number 54. Westport, CT: Greenwood Press.

Kopp, J.R., H. Alexander, R.H. Turocy, M.G. Levrini, D.M. Lichtman. 1986. The use of lumbar extension in evaluation and treatment of patients with acute herniated nucleus pulposus: A preliminary report. *Clinical Orthopaedics* 202 (January): 211-218.

Korzybski, Alfred H. 1990. *Alfred Korzybski: Collected writings 1920-1950.* Collected and arranged by M. Kendig. Englewood, NJ: Institute of General Semantics.

―――. 1933, 1994. *Science and sanity: An introduction to non-aristotelian systems and General Semantics.* Fifth Edition. Englewood, NJ: International Non-Aristotelian Library, Institute of General Semantics.

Krämer, Jürgen et al. Trans. K.H. Mueller, et al. 1990. *Intervertebral disk disease: Causes, diagnosis, treatment and prophylaxis.* New York: Georg Thieme Verlag Stuttgart.

Krucoff, Carol. 2000. "Got no time for serious fitness training? The long and short of it. Exercise: Researchers now say that little 'sparks' of activity throughout the day can offer health benefits." *Los Angeles Times,* 12/04: S1, S8.

Kuslich, S., C. L. Ulstrom and C. J. Michael. 1991. The tissue origin of low back pain and sciatica: A report of pain response to tissue stimulation during operations on the lumbar spine using local anesthesia. *Ortho Clinics of North America* 22 (2):181-187.

Langer, Ellen J. 1989. *Mindfulness.* Reading, MA: Addison-Wesley.

Laslett, Mark. 1996. *Mechanical diagnosis and therapy: The upper limb.* N.p.

Laslett, Mark and Paula van Wijman. 1999. Low back and referred pain: Diagnosis and a proposed new system of classification. *New Zealand Journal of Physiotherapy* 27: 5-14.

Laszlo, Ervin, Robert Artigiani, Allan Combs, and Vilmos Csanyi. 1996. *Changing visions: Human cognitive maps—past, present, and future.* Westport, CT: Praeger.

Licht, Sidney. 1978. History. In *Therapeutic exercise.* Third Edition. Ed. John V. Basmajian, 1-42. Baltimore: Williams & Wilkins.

Liebenson, Craig, ed. 1996. *Rehabilitation of the spine: A practitioner's manual.* Baltimore: Williams & Wilkins.

Liebman, Michael. 1979. *Neuroanatomy made easy and understandable.* Baltimore: University Park Press.

"Life-saving prescription." 2000. *The back letter* 15 (11): 132.

Livingston, Michael. n.d. *Back aid: Your guide to care of the back.* Philadelphia: George F. Stickley Company.

Long, Audrey. 1995. The centralization phenomenon: Its usefulness as a predictor of outcome in conservative treatment of chronic low back pain (a pilot study). *Spine* 20 (23): 2513-2521.

Low back pain care. 1999. Submitted by the Group Health Physical and Occupational Therapy Service. *The McKenzie Journal* 7 (1): 34-36.

Macdonald, Patrick. 1989. *The Alexander Technique as I see it.* Brighton, UK: Rahula Books.

Macnab, Ian. 1977. *Backache.* Baltimore: Williams & Wilkins.

Magner, George. 1995. *Chiropractic: the victim's perspective.* Ed. Stephen Barrett. Buffalo, NY: Prometheus Books.

Maitland, Geoffrey D. 1987. The Maitland principle: Assessment, examination, and treatment by passive movement. In *Physical therapy of the low back,* ed. Lance T. Twomey and James R. Taylor, 135-155. New York: Churchill Livingstone.

————. 1986. *Vertebral manipulation.* Fifth Edition. London: Butterworth Heinemann.

Major sciatica treatment proves ineffective in landmark randomized trial. 1999. *The Back Letter* 14 (3): 25.

Mandal, A.C. Balanced sitting posture on forward sloping seat. Available at http://www.acmandal.com/

Marken, Richard S. 1992. *Mind readings: Experimental studies of purpose.* Chapel Hill, NC: Control Systems Group/New View Publications.

Martin, Robert Manatt. 1975. *The gravity guiding system.* Pasadena, CA: Gravity Guidance, Inc.

Mathews, Ann. 1984. *Implications for education in the work of F. M. Alexander: An exploratory project in a public school classroom.* Master's Thesis. Available from Institute for Research, Development & Education in the Alexander Technique, 74 MacDougal St. NY, NY 10012.

Mathews, Troup H. 1991. Blessed helicity. *Direction: A journal of the Alexander Technique* 1 (8): 308-314.

McCombe, P.F., J.C.T. Fairbank,, B.C. Cockersole, et al. 1989. Reproducibility of physical signs in low-back pain. *Spine* 14:9, 908-918.

McGregor, Rob Roy. 1982. *EEVeTeCh.* New York: Houghton Mifflin.

McKenzie, Robin. 1999. Re: Understanding centralisation. *The McKenzie Journal* 7 (3): 6-8.

————. 1997a. *Treat your own back.* 7th Ed. Waikanae, NZ: Spinal Publications.

————. 1997b. *Treat your own neck.* 3rd Ed. Waikanae, NZ: Spinal Publications.

————. 1990. *The cervical and thoracic spine: Mechanical diagnosis and therapy.* Waikanae, NZ: Spinal Publications.

————. 1981. *The lumbar spine: Mechanical diagnosis and therapy.* Waikanae, NZ: Spinal Publications.

McKenzie, Robin with Craig Kubey. 2000. *7 steps to a pain-free life: How to rapidly relieve back and neck pain using the McKenzie method.* New York: E.P. Dutton.

McKenzie, Robin and Stephen May. 2000. *The human extremities: Mechanical diagnosis & therapy.* Waikanae, New Zealand: Spinal Publications.

Melzack, Ronald and Patrick D. Wall. 1982. *The challenge of pain.* New York: Basic Books.

Mennell, John McM. 1960. *Back pain: Diagnosis and treatment using manipulative techniques.* Boston: Little, Brown.

Merskey, H. and N. Bogduk. 1994. *Classification of chronic pain*, Second Edition. IASP Task Force on Taxonomy. Seattle: IASP Press.

Moffat, Marilyn and Steve Vickery. 1999. *The American Physical Therapy Association book of body maintenance and repair.* New York: Henry Holt.

Montagu, Ashley. 1986. *Touching: The human significance of the skin.* Third Edition. New York: Harper & Row.

———. 1981. *Growing Young.* New York: McGraw-Hill.

———. 1951. *On being intelligent.* Westport, CT: Greenwood Press.

Neev, Elan Z. 1993. *Wholistic healing.* Fifth edition. Beverly Hills, CA: Ageless Books.

New UK back pain guidelines. 1997. *The Back Letter* 12 (1).

OSHA (Occupational Safety & Health Administration). Ergonomics. http://www.osha-slc.gov/SLTC/ergonomics/

Paris, Stanley V. 1989. The Paris approach. In *Postgraduate advances in the evaluation and treatment of low back dysfunction.* Berryville, VA: Forum Medicum.

———. 1979. *The spine: Etiology and treatment of dysfunction including joint manipulation.* Bound course notes.

Pert, Candace B. 1997. *The molecules of emotion: Why you feel the way you feel.* New York: Scribner.

Peter, Laurence J. 1979. *Peter's people.* New York: William Morrow.

———. 1977. *Peter's quotations: Ideas for our time.* New York: Quill, William Morrow.

Pheasant, Stephen and David Stubbs. 1992. Back pain in nurses: Epidemiology and risk asssessment. *Applied Ergonomics* 23 (4): 226-232.

Pople, I.K., H.B. Griffith. 1994. Prediction of an extruded fragment in lumbar disc patients from clinical presentations. *Spine* 19(2): 156-158.

Powers, William T. 1998. *Making sense of behavior: The meaning of control.* New Canaan, CT: Benchmark Publications.

———. 1992. *Living control systems II: Selected papers of William T. Powers.* Gravel Switch, Kentucky: The Control Systems Group.

———. 1989. *Living control systems: Selected papers of William T. Powers.* Gravel Switch, Kentucky: The Control Systems Group.

———. 1973. *Behavior: The control of perception.* New York: Aldine De Gruyter.

Prevalence of back pain — by quality of study. June 1999. *The Back Letter* 14 (6).

Pula, Robert P. 2000. *A General Semantics glossary: Pula's guide for the perplexed.* Concord, CA: International Society for General Semantics.

Rath, Wayne W. and Jean Duffy Rath. 1992. Prevention of musculoskeletal injury. In *Prevention practice: Strategies for physical therapy and occupational therapy*, ed. Jeffrey Rothman and Ruth Levine, 74-114. Philadelphia: W.B. Saunders.

Rickover, Robert M. 1988. *Fitness without stress: A guide to the Alexander Technique*. Portland, OR: Metamorphous Press.

Rizzo, J. A., et al. 1998. The labor productivity effects of chronic backache in the United States, Medical Care 36(10):1471-1488.

Robertson, Richard J. 1998. Control theory. In *Concise encyclopedia of psychology*, Second Edition, Abridged. Ed. Raymond J. Corsini and Alan J. Auerback, 170-171. New York: John Wiley & Sons.

Robertson, Richard J. and William T. Powers, eds. 1990. *Introduction to modern psychology: The control-theory view*. Gravel Switch, Kentucky: The Control Systems Group.

Rossi, Ernest Lawrence with David Nimmons. 1991. *The 20-minute break*. Los Angeles: Jeremy P. Tarcher.

Rossi, Ernest Lawrence. 1986. *The psychobiology of mind-body healing*. New York: W.W. Norton.

Rosten, Leo. 1972. *Leo Rosten's treasury of Jewish quotations*. New York: Bantam.

———. 1968. *The joys of Yiddish*. New York: Pocket Books.

Royal College of General Practitioners. 1996. *Clinical guidelines for the management of acute low back pain*. London: RCGP. Available at http://www.rcgp.org.uk/college/activity/qualclin/guides/backpain/index.htm

Runkel, Philip J. 1990. *Casting nets and testing specimens: Two grand methods of psychology*. New York: Praeger.

Sacks, Oliver W. 1987. *The man who mistook his wife for a hat and other clinical tales*. New York: Harper & Row.

———. 1984. *A leg to stand on*. London: Duckworth.

Samanta, Ash and Jo Beardsley. April 24, 1999. "Low back pain: which is the best way forward?" *British Medical Journal* 3 (18): 1122-3.

Sarno, John E. 1991. *Healing back pain: The mind-body connection*. New York: Warner Books.

Sharaf, Myron. 1983. *Fury on earth: A biography of Wilhelm Reich*. New York: St. Martins Press/Marek.

Sherrington, Charles S. 1953. *Man on his nature*. Second Edition. New York: Doubleday Anchor.

————. *The endeavor of Jean Fernal.* 1946. Cambridge, UK: Cambridge University Press.

Smallheiser, Marvin.1988. William Chen on T'ai Chi Ch'uan for fighting. *Ta'i Chi: The leading international journal of T'ai Chi Ch'uan* 12 (5): 2-3,19.

Snook, Stover H., Barbara S. Webster, Raymond W. McGorry, Maxwell T. Fogleman and Kathleen B. McCann. 1998. The Reduction of chronic nonspecific low back pain through the control of early morning lumbar flexion: A randomized controlled trial. *Spine* 23 (Dec. 1): 2601-2607.

Snorrason, Egill. 1965. Exercise for healthy persons. In *Therapeutic exercise*. Second Edition, Revised. Ed. Sidney Licht, 896-911. New Haven: Elizabeth Licht.

Sontag, Jerry, ed. 1996. *Curiosity recaptured: Exploring ways we think and move.* San Francisco: Mornum Time Press.

Speads, Carola. 1978. *Breathing: The ABC's.* New York: Harper Collophon.

Spinal overload. November 1999. *The Back Letter* 14 (11).

Spratt, K.F., T.R. Lehmann, J.N. Weinstein, H. A. Sayre. 1990. A new approach to the low back physical examination, behavioral assessment of mechanical signs. *Spine* 15(2).

Stankovic, R., O. Johnell. 1995. Conservative treatment of acute low back pain: A 5-year follow-up study of two methods of treatment. *Spine* 20 (4).

————. 1990. Conservative treatment of acute low back pain; A prospective randomized trial: McKenzie method versus patient education in "Mini back school." *Spine* 15 (2).

Staring, Jeroen.1997. *The first 43 years of the life of F. Matthias Alexander. Volume 2.* Nijmegen, The Netherlands.

Steering Committee for the Workshop on Work-Related Musculoskeletal Injuries. 1999. *Work-related musculoskeletal disorders*. Washington, DC: National Academy Press.

Stevens, Chris.1990, 1995. *Towards a physiology of the F.M. Alexander Technique: A record of work in progress.* London: STAT Books.

Stoddard, Alan. 1979. *The back: Relief from pain.* New York: Arco.

Stone, Justin F. 1996. *T'ai Chi Chih: Joy thru movement.* Fort Yates, ND: Good Karma Publishing.

Thompson, Kay. 1987. *NYSEPH presents Kay Thompson, D.D.S.: Therapeutic uses of language.* (Tapes of Course). New York: The New York Milton H. Erickson Society for Psychotherapy and Hypnosis.

Trager, Milton with Cathy Guadagno. *Trager mentastics: Movement as a way to agelessness.* Barrytown, NY: Station Hill.

Tucker, W. E. 1960. *Active alerted posture*. London: Livingstone.

Twomey, Lance T. and James R. Taylor, eds. 1987. *Physical therapy of the low back. Vol. 13 – Clinics in physical therapy*. New York: Churchill Livingstone.

Uderman, B.E., et al. 2000. Can an educational booklet change behavior and pain in chronic low back pain patients (abstract). *McKenzie Journal* 8 (3): 55.

Van Wijman, Paula M. 1994. The use of repeated movements in the McKenzie method of spinal examination. Reprinted 1995 in *The McKenzie Institute, USA Newsletter* 3 (2). Originally published in *Modern manual therapy of the vertebral column*, Second Edition, ed. Boyling & Palastanga, Chapter 42.

Von Durkheim, Karlfried Graf. 1962, 1977. *Hara: The vital centre of man*. Translated by Sylvia-Monica von Kospoth in collaboration with Estelle R. Healey. London: Unwin.

Waddell, Gordon. 1998. *The back pain revolution*. Edinburgh: Churchill Livingstone.

Waddington, C. H. 1977. *Tools for thought: How to understand and apply the latest scientific techniques of problem solving*. New York: Basic.

Wall, Patrick. 2000. *Pain: The science of suffering*. New York: Columbia University Press.

Ward, Milton. 1977. *The brilliant function of pain: A yogic understanding of pain*. New York: Optimus Books.

Werneke, Mark, D. Hart and D. Cook. 1999. A descriptive study of the centralization phenomenon: A prospective analysis. *Spine* 24: 676-683.

Whatmore, George B. and Daniel R. Kohli. 1968. Dysponesis: A neurophysiological factor in functional disorders. *Behavioral Science* 13(2).

Whitehead, Alfred North. 1925, 1948. *Science and the modern world: Lowell lectures, 1925*. New York: Pelican Mentor.

Wassell, James T, Lytt I. Gardner, Douglas P. Landsittel, Janet J. Johnston, Janet M. Johnston. 2000. A prospective study of back belts for prevention of back pain and injury. *JAMA* 284 (21): 2727-2732 (Dec. 6).

Westfeldt, Lulie. 1964, 1986. *F. Matthias Alexander: The man and his work*. Long Beach, CA: Centerline Press.

Whyte, Lancelot Law. 1950. *The next development in man*. New York: Mentor Books.

Williams, M.M., J. A. Hawley, R. A. McKenzie, P. M. Van Wijmen. 1991. A comparison of the effects of two sitting postures on back and referred pain. *Spine* 116 (10): 1185-1191.

Yesudian, Selvarajan and Elisabeth Haich. 1953, 1976. *Yoga and health*. London: Unwin.

INDEX

About the Author

Bruce I. Kodish, Ph.D., P.T., has worked as a physical therapist since 1981, with wide-ranging experience in hospitals, nursing homes, rehabilitation centers, orthopedic clinics, home care and private practice.

A certified teaching member of the American Society for the Alexander Technique and certified in Mechanical Diagnosis and Therapy (MDT), he has studied a variety of posture-movement education and therapy approaches with emphasis on back and neck problems. In his private practice, Dr. Kodish, whose Ph.D. is in General Semantics (applied epistemology) provides his unique synthesis of posture-movement therapy and posture-movement education.

He is co-author, with his wife Susan Presby Kodish, Ph.D., a psychologist, of *Drive Yourself Sane: Using The Uncommon Sense of General Semantics.* They continue to write about and teach General Semantics in relation to a variety of applications. Both are dedicated to the goal of applying and helping others to apply a scientific attitude in everyday life.

Order Form

Check your local bookstore to obtain additional copies. If you prefer to order directly from us by mail, you can copy this form and pay by check or money order. All major credit cards are accepted online with secure ordering at **www.backpainsolutions.net**

Name:_____

Address: _____

City: _____ State/Province: _____

Country: _____ Zip/Postal Code: _____

Phone:_____ Fax: _____

Email Address:_____

Please ship the following books:

	Price (US $)		Quantity	Subtotal
Back Pain Solutions: *How to Help Yourself with Posture-Movement Therapy and Education* 2001, 320 pages ISBN 0-9700664-5-7	20.00	x	—————	—————
Drive Yourself Sane: *Using the Uncommon Sense of General Semantics* 2nd. Ed. 2001, 236 pages ISBN 0-9700664-6-5	18.00	x	—————	—————

In California, please add Sales Tax. ————————

Shipping & Handling:
US: add $ 4.00 for first book and $ 2.00 for each additional book; Canada/Mexico: add $5.00 for first book and $3.00 for each additional book. Other International: add $9.00 for first book and $ 5.00 for each additional book.

————————

Make check/money order payable and mail to:
      Extensional Publishing
        P. O. Box 50490
     Pasadena, CA 91115-0490

Total: ————————